Multiple Sclerosis - Genetics, Disease Mechanisms and Clinical Developments

Edited by Uday Kishore and Abhishek Shastri

Published in London, United Kingdom

Multiple Sclerosis - Genetics, Disease Mechanisms and Clinical Developments
http://dx.doi.org/10.5772/intechopen.98110
Edited by Uday Kishore and Abhishek Shastri

Contributors
Valentina Ignatova, Bilyana Mihaylova, Silviya Cherninkova, Arthi Balasundaram, Mohan Krishna Ghanta, Omar Deeb, Sawsan Salameh, Afnan Atallah, Uday Kishore, Abhishek Shastri, Raphiq Ibrahim, Iesha Singh

First published in London, United Kingdom, 2024 by IntechOpen
IntechOpen is the global imprint of INTECHOPEN LIMITED, registered in England and Wales, registration number: 11086078, 5 Princes Gate Court, London, SW7 2QJ, United Kingdom

British Library Cataloguing-in-Publication Data
A catalogue record for this book is available from the British Library

Additional hard and PDF copies can be obtained from orders@intechopen.com

Multiple Sclerosis - Genetics, Disease Mechanisms and Clinical Developments
Edited by Uday Kishore and Abhishek Shastri
p. cm.
Print ISBN 978-1-80356-008-3
Online ISBN 978-1-80356-009-0
eBook (PDF) ISBN 978-1-80356-010-6

For EU product safety concerns:
IN TECH d.o.o., Prolaz Marije Krucifikse Kozulić 3, 51000 Rijeka, Croatia,
info@intechopen.com or visit our website at intechopen.com.

Meet the editors

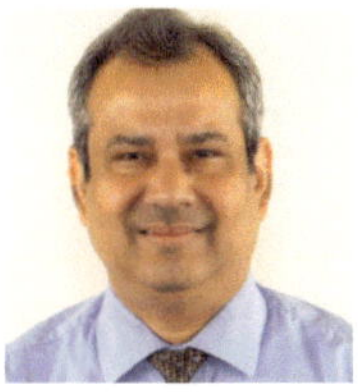

Prof. Uday Kishore is a passionate and translational researcher, an inspiring, engaging, and inclusive teacher, an academic leader with a wide research network internationally and across higher education, charity, pharma, and biotech sectors, and an inventor of biologics for clinical trials. He is a teacher and a scientist with a special interest in innate immunity. He was the founder-director of the Centre for Infection, Immunity and Disease Mechanisms, Brunel University London. He obtained a BSc from S.P. Jain College, Sasaram, Bihar, India; an MSc from Hindu College, Delhi University; and a Ph.D. from the Department of Zoology, University of Delhi and CSIR Institute of Genomics and Integrative Biology, Delhi, India. After spending a year at the Salk Institute for Biological Studies, La Jolla, California, USA, Dr. Kishore moved to the University of Oxford for the major part of his post-doctoral training, first at the MRC Immunochemistry Unit, Department of Biochemistry, and then at the Weatherall Institute of Molecular Medicine, John Radcliffe Hospital. He is the recipient of fellowships from NASA (USA), Wellcome Trust (UK), and Alexander Humboldt Foundation (Germany). He is the recipient of the MRC Investigator Prize, European Commission Young Scientist Prize, and Mother Teresa Excellence Award. He is also a fellow of the Royal Society of Biology UK (FRSB) and the Royal College of Pathologists (FRCPath London). Dr. Kishore holds several adjunct, visiting, and honorary professorial positions nationally and internationally. He has authored nearly 300 research papers, book chapters, patents, and books. His research focuses on how innate immunity plays a crucial role in human health and disease. He has extensive experience researching autoimmune diseases such as systemic lupus erythematosus and myasthenia gravis.

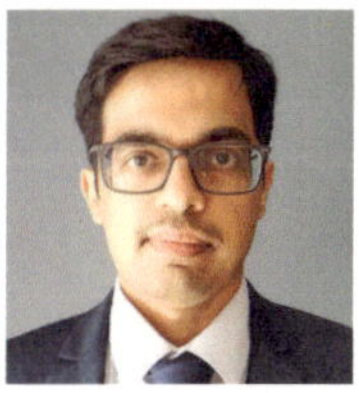

Dr. Abhishek Shastri is a consultant psychiatrist for a busy London dementia service. He graduated with a degree in medicine from Rajiv Gandhi University of Health Sciences, Bangalore, India, in 2010. He obtained a postgraduate diploma in psychiatry from Cardiff University, Wales, and secured an MPhil in Neuroinflammation from Brunel University London. He then trained in Bournemouth and Poole where he obtained membership in the Royal College of Psychiatrists and subsequently completed his higher specialist training in Kensington and Chelsea and Westminster. Dr. Shastri has published numerous articles and book chapters on neuroinflammation and dementias. He is a clinical and educational supervisor for core and higher trainees in psychiatry for the Health Education London training scheme.

Contents

Preface

Multiple sclerosis (MS) is a neurological condition that affects the central nervous system (CNS). A diagnosis of MS can mean a lifelong illness that ranges from mild to severely debilitating. There is no known cure for the disease. Over the years, extensive research has been carried out to fully understand its etiology and pathogenesis, alongside robust clinical trials being conducted to develop effective therapeutic avenues. Research, as well as clinical trials, continue to take place across the world to help find a cure for MS. There is a very close interplay of immunological mechanisms in the development and progression of MS.

This book brings together the latest, cutting-edge research findings along with expert commentary on epidemiology, genetics, biomarkers, etiology, pathogenesis, immunology, neuroimaging, and clinical treatment modalities of this chronic inflammatory disease affecting the CNS. The book begins with an introductory chapter about MS that provides an in-depth understanding of the latest developments in disease-modifying therapies, stem-cell therapies, and neuroimaging. The next chapter delves into the interesting sphere of biomarkers for MS that may be helpful as diagnostic and prognostic markers of treatment. This is followed by a chapter that explores the impact of genetics and environmental and lifestyle factors that are of significant importance in MS. We then move on to an excellent piece of original research on ocular imaging in patients, and its usefulness in understanding the progression of MS. Following this, we examine the potential and role of artificial intelligence in the management of MS and in improving MS research. In the next section, we examine the impact of cognition and brain health on MS disease progression. The book ends with an in-depth assessment of the role of innate immunity in the pathogenesis of MS to help understand the disease and inform treatment modalities. We hope that readers find the book useful in helping improve their understanding of MS, as well as in furthering their interest in MS research and its clinical aspects.

Uday Kishore, Ph.D., FHEA, FRSB, FRCPath
Department of Veterinary Medicine,
UAE University,
Al Ain, United Arab Emirates

Abhishek Shastri, MBBS, Mphil, MRCPsych
Central and North West London NHS Foundation Trust,
London, United Kingdom

Section 1

Avant-Garde in Multiple Sclerosis

Chapter 1

Introductory Chapter: State-of-the-Art Developments in Multiple Sclerosis

Abhishek Shastri and Uday Kishore

1. Introduction

Multiple sclerosis (MS) is an immune-mediated, progressive neurological disease with a heterogeneous course of illness. The symptoms can vary from person-to-person and can include problems with balance, vision, movements of limbs and sensation, cognitive deficits, gait difficulties and bladder dysfunction [1]. According to the World Health Organisation Atlas of MS report in 2020, 2.8 million people were reported to be living with MS worldwide, which is about 1 in 3000 people [1]. MS is nearly twice as more common in females (69%) as compared to males (31%); the majority of diagnosis are made between the ages of 20 and 50 years, although MS also occurs in young children and older adults [1]. More recently, Epstein-Barr virus (EBV) has emerged as an important link in epidemiological studies with patients infected with EBV having a higher risk of developing MS [2]. Smoking and diet also play a significant role in MS. A recent UK biobank study of nearly 8000 people showed that cessation of smoking was related to reduced deterioration in motor function and mobility in MS [3]. A diet that avoids processed foods, gluten, lectins and casein, and a diet that contains low-saturated fats were also found to be helpful in reducing fatigue in MS patients [4].

MS pathogenesis is considered to be autoimmune in nature and myelin proteins have been studied in detail and used to induce MS-like disease features in animal models, termed as experimental autoimmune encephalomyelitis. Some of the other key pathological features include neuroinflammation, breakdown of blood-brain barrier and gliosis. Both innate and adaptive immune systems play a role in MS disease pathogenesis [5]. Taking forward the recent finding of higher risk with EBV infection, a mechanistic link has been found that could possibly explain the role of EBV. Molecular mimicry[1] between a transcription factor of EBV, termed as EBV nuclear antigen 1 (EBNA1), and CNS glial cell adhesion molecule (GlialCAM), was demonstrated. Immunisation with EBNA1 in mouse model of MS was found to exacerbate the disease. The same study also found that MS patients had prevalence of anti-EBNA1 and anti-GlialCAM antibodies [6]. Latest research on myelin regeneration in a zebra fish model found that some oligodendrocytes (cells that produce myelin) survive demyelination in MS and go on to produce aberrant and

[1] Molecular mimicry refers to the immunological and structural similarities between molecules found in pathogens and host cells, which leads to immune response in the host. Molecular mimicry is considered to play a significant role in autoimmune diseases.

mistargeted new myelin, as compared to new oligodendrocytes that are produced after demyelination [7].

Clinically, there are four different types of MS, namely: (i) relapsing-remitting MS (RRMS), which is the most common type that is characterised by exacerbations of illness followed by partial or complete recovery; (ii) primary progressive MS (PPMS) characterised by progressive worsening of neurological function or disability from the onset of illness; (iii) secondary progressive MS (SPMS) characterised by initial relapsing-remitting course followed by progressive increase in neurological function or disability; and (iv) clinically isolated syndrome (CIS) characterised by monophasic or first episode of neurological dysfunction associated with demyelination and inflammation in the central nervous system (CNS) occurring in a patient not known to have MS [8]. Treatment involves a multi-disciplinary approach due to the varying symptoms that occur in MS. Hence, different professionals are involved such as neurologist, specialist nurse, physiotherapist, occupational therapist, urologist, rehabilitation specialists in a multi-pronged approach to manage MS. The mainstay of medical management is oral and monoclonal antibody therapies called as disease modifying therapies (DMTs).

2. Latest in DMT research

DMTs are available to MS patients in oral, injection and infusion forms. Mechanism of action for DMTs includes immunomodulation or immunosuppression affecting lymphocyte number, lymphocyte proliferation, lymphocyte trafficking or cytokine production (**Figure 1**) [9]. Thus, DMTs reduce neuroinflammation in CNS, and prevent relapses and new lesion formation. For RRMS, there are over a dozen DMTs that have been licenced for use; for PPMS, ocrelizumab, which is a monoclonal antibody against CD20 antigen expressed on B cells, has been recently licenced for use; for CIS, preparations of interferon beta, which reduce secretion of proinflammatory cytokines, and T cell trafficking in CNS or glatiramer acetate, which stimulates myelin protein and T cell modulation, are used [9, 10]. Some of the other DMTs used in MS treatment are natalizumab (monoclonal antibody, α4 integrin receptor antagonist that reduces T cell and leucocyte migration across blood-brain barrier); cladribine (anti-metabolite that causes depletion in T and B cells), teriflunomide (inhibitor of pyrimidine synthesis that causes reduction in lymphocytes), etc. [9, 10]. Specific mechanisms of action are poorly understood and DMTs are associated with a range of unwanted side effects and safety concerns that require regular and robust monitoring. Some mild side effects include flu-like symptoms or gastrointestinal tract upset; however, serious side effects include cardiac arrhythmias, malignancy and liver damage [9].

3. Latest in stem cell transplantation therapies in MS

Autologous haematopoietic stem cell transplantation (aHSCT) is a newer type of treatment for MS. Guidelines recommend that aHSCT is offered to those patients with highly active RRMS where DMTs have been ineffective [11, 12]. In short, the first step in aHSCT involves chemotherapy and growth factor such as granulocyte colony-stimulating factor so that stem cells move from bone marrow into blood stream from where the stem cells are harvested and then frozen.

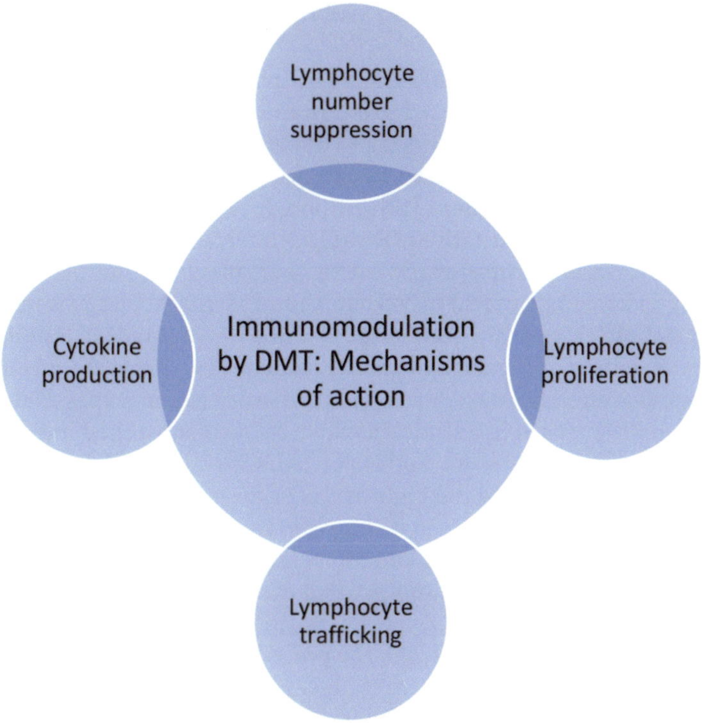

Figure 1.
Mechanism of action for DMTs in MS. These include immunomodulation by suppression of lymphocyte numbers, modulating lymphocyte proliferation and trafficking and production of cytokines. Adapted from [9]. Abbreviations: DMT: Disease-modifying treatment; MS: Multiple sclerosis.

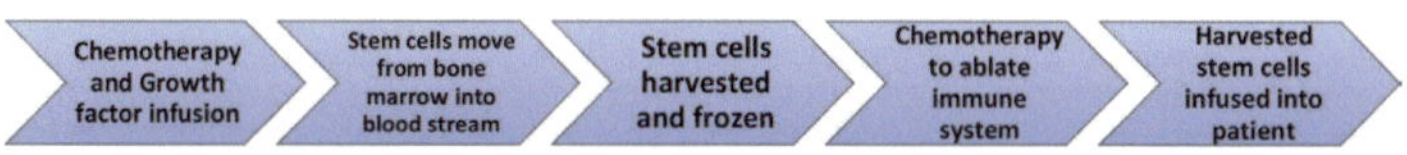

Figure 2.
Flow diagram to show process of aHSCT treatment in MS. A patient with MS first undergoes chemotherapy and growth factor infusion so that stem cells move from bone marrow into the blood stream. Then, stem cells are harvested and frozen for later use. Next, chemotherapy is done to ablate the existing aberrant immune system of patient with MS, following which the harvested stem cells are infused back into the patient. Abbreviation: aHSCT: Autologous haematopoietic stem cell transplantation; MS: Multiple sclerosis.

Following this, chemotherapy is done so that the immune system is ablated or 'wiped out'. Next, the harvested stem cells are infused into the patient, for reconstitution of the immune system (**Figure 2**). The entire process of preparation, harvesting and reconditioning of immune system can take 3–4 months, which then requires long-term follow-up clinically [13, 14]. A Phase 3 randomised controlled trial comparing aHSCT with older DMTs showed that aHSCT is effective in RRMS [15] but there are no studies comparing efficacy of aHSCT with newer DMTs [13]. Another type of stem cell transplantation technique that is also finding ground in MS is called autologous mesenchymal stem cell transplantation (AMSCT). MSCs are non-haematopoietic stromal stem cells found in the bone marrow. Phase 2 randomised controlled clinical trials against placebo have found AMSCT to be safe in MS patients [16] and also to be beneficial in PPMS by improving cognition and reducing relapses [17].

4. Latest research on neuroimaging and biomarkers in MS

Magnetic resonance imaging (MRI) is the mainstay of diagnosing MS radiologically. Gadolinium is a key marker used to study and phenotype MS, and it acts as a marker for neuroinflammatory lesions and blood-brain barrier breakdown. It also aids in the diagnostic process to some extent by helping in monitoring disease progression or efficacy of treatment [18]. Although conventional MRIs are useful in qualitative information, quantitative MRIs (QMRI; which involve disentangling the source of signal variation in images and use mathematical or computational modelling) are being increasingly useful in MS clinics and research. QMRI is more specific for studying and differentiating between grey and white matter MS lesions and for detecting the extent of myelin and axonal damage [19]. Recently, unsupervised machine-based learning has been developed to identify MS subtypes. Dataset for over 6000 MS patients were used in a study, in which MS was sub-typed into cortex-led, normal appearing white matter-led and lesion led. Clinical correlation showed that patients with lesion-led MS had the highest risk of disability and relapse rate. Patients in this subtype also showed increased response to treatment [20].

Discovering effective molecular biomarkers is also an extensive area for on-going research. There is good evidence to suggest that early detection and treatment of MS has a better prognosis [21]. Thus, the quest is to find markers that are found in the early stages of illness, or even perhaps in the preceding stage of appearance of clinical features in MS. At present, CSF analysis for IgG index and oligoclonal bands are used in supporting a diagnosis of MS [22, 23]. Other known CSF biomarkers include neurofilament light chain [24], chemokine CXC motif ligand 13 (CCL13) [25], osteopontin [26] and matrix metallopeptidase 9 [27]. Progress is also being made in identifying serum markers. A recent study found two proteins, oncostatin M and hepatocyte growth factor, to be associated with MS in comparison with healthy controls [28]. The same study also found that plasma CCL20 and CCL11 were associated with MS disease duration and progression [28].

5. Perspectives

MS is a disease with a complex heterogeneity in clinical presentation, neuroinflammatory lesions, imaging and treatment response. This leads to challenges in various stages of MS disease pathogenesis, for example in the initial diagnostic stage of varying symptomatology and neuroimaging, as well as in identifying appropriate treatment with DMTs. For MS patients, the degree of disability and prognosis varies and is difficult to predict. All of these throw up opportunities for research in MS, such as identifying and classifying MS lesions, predicting response to therapy, improving neuroimaging accuracy and its usefulness in predicting outcome, biomarkers for early detection and for detecting response to treatment. This introductory chapter, and indeed the entire book, is intended to stimulate interest in these areas of MS research and to serve as a good starting point to ensure readers can get maximum benefit from reading the upcoming chapters. Several such wonderful areas of research are covered in this book, which range from biomarkers, genetic and lifestyle factors affecting MS, to imaging techniques and innate immune mechanisms in MS. We hope you find this book a useful tool in enhancing your knowledge and understanding of MS, as well as to stimulate your interest in the different spheres of MS research.

Author details

Abhishek Shastri[1*] and Uday Kishore[2]

1 Central and North West London NHS Foundation Trust, London, United Kingdom

2 Department of Veterinary Medicine, UAE University, Al Ain, United Arab Emirates

*Address all correspondence to: abhishek.shastri@nhs.net

References

[1] The Multiple Sclerosis International Federation, Atlas of MS, 3rd Edition (September 2020)

[2] Bjornevik K, Cortese M, Healy BC, Kuhle J, Mina MJ, Leng Y, et al. Longitudinal analysis reveals high prevalence of Epstein-Barr virus associated with multiple sclerosis. Science. 2022;**375**(6578):296-301

[3] Rodgers J, Friede T, Vonberg FW, Constantinescu CS, Coles A, Chataway J, et al. The impact of smoking cessation on multiple sclerosis disease progression. Brain. 2022;**145**(4):1368-1378

[4] Wahls TL, Titcomb TJ, Bisht B, Eyck PT, Rubenstein LM, Carr LJ, et al. Impact of the swank and Wahls elimination dietary interventions on fatigue and quality of life in relapsing-remitting multiple sclerosis: The WAVES randomized parallel-arm clinical trial. Multiple Sclerosis Journal – Experimental, Translational and Clinical. 2021;**7**(3):20552173211035399

[5] Loma I, Heyman R. Multiple sclerosis: Pathogenesis and treatment. Current Neuropharmacology. 2011 Sep;**9**(3):409-416

[6] Lanz TV, Brewer RC, Ho PP, Moon J, Jude KM, Fernandez D, et al. Clonally expanded B cells in multiple sclerosis bind EBV EBNA1 and GlialCAM. Nature. 2022;**603**(7900):321-327

[7] Neely SA, Williamson JM, Klingseisen A, Zoupi L, Early JJ, Williams A, et al. New oligodendrocytes exhibit more abundant and accurate myelin regeneration than those that survive demyelination. Nature Neuroscience. 2022;**25**(4):415-420

[8] Lublin FD, Coetzee T, Cohen JA, Marrie RA, Thompson AJ. International Advisory Committee on Clinical Trials in MS. The 2013 clinical course descriptors for multiple sclerosis: A clarification. Neurology. 2020;**94**(24):1088-1092

[9] De Angelis F, John NA, Brownlee WJ. Disease-modifying therapies for multiple sclerosis. BMJ. 2018;**363**:k4674

[10] Wingerchuk DM, Weinshenker BG. Disease modifying therapies for relapsing multiple sclerosis. BMJ. 2016;**354**:i3518

[11] Treatment algorithm for Multiple Sclerosis Disease-Modifying therapies. Available from: https://www.england.nhs.uk/commissioning/wp-content/uploads/sites/12/2019/03/Treatment-Algorithm-for-Multiple-Sclerosis-Disease-Modifying-Therapies-08-03-2019-1.pdf

[12] Sharrack B, Saccardi R, Alexander T, Badoglio M, Burman J, Farge D, et al. Autologous haematopoietic stem cell transplantation and other cellular therapy in multiple sclerosis and immune-mediated neurological diseases: Updated guidelines and recommendations from the EBMT autoimmune diseases working party (ADWP) and the joint accreditation committee of EBMT and ISCT (JACIE). Bone Marrow Transplantation. 2020;**55**(2):283-306

[13] Sharrack B, Petrie J, Coles A, Snowden JA. Is stem cell transplantation safe and effective in multiple sclerosis? BMJ. 2022;**377**:e061514-2020-061514

[14] Muraro PA, Martin R, Mancardi GL, Nicholas R, Sormani MP, Saccardi R. Autologous haematopoietic stem cell

transplantation for treatment of multiple sclerosis. Nature Reviews. Neurology. 2017;**13**(7):391-405

[15] Burt RK, Han X, Quigley K, Helenowski IB, Balabanov R. Real-world application of autologous hematopoietic stem cell transplantation in 507 patients with multiple sclerosis. Journal of Neurology. 2022;**269**(5):2513-2526

[16] Uccelli A, Laroni A, Ali R, Battaglia MA, Blinkenberg M, Brundin L, et al. Safety, tolerability, and activity of mesenchymal stem cells versus placebo in multiple sclerosis (MESEMS): A phase 2, randomised, double-blind crossover trial. Lancet Neurology. 2021;**20**(11):917-929

[17] Petrou P, Kassis I, Levin N, Paul F, Backner Y, Benoliel T, et al. Beneficial effects of autologous mesenchymal stem cell transplantation in active progressive multiple sclerosis. Brain. 2020;**143**(12):3574-3588

[18] Wattjes MP, Ciccarelli O, Reich DS, Banwell B, de Stefano N, Enzinger C, et al. 2021 MAGNIMS-CMSC-NAIMS consensus recommendations on the use of MRI in patients with multiple sclerosis. Lancet Neurology. 2021;**20**(8):653-670

[19] Granziera C, Wuerfel J, Barkhof F, Calabrese M, De Stefano N, Enzinger C, et al. Quantitative magnetic resonance imaging towards clinical application in multiple sclerosis. Brain. 2021;**144**(5):1296-1311

[20] Eshaghi A, Young AL, Wijeratne PA, Prados F, Arnold DL, Narayanan S, et al. Identifying multiple sclerosis subtypes using unsupervised machine learning and MRI data. Nature Communications. 2021;**12**(1):2078-021-22265-2

[21] Meca-Lallana JE, Casanova B, Rodriguez-Antiguedad A, Eichau S, Izquierdo G, Duran C, et al. Consensus on early detection of disease progression in patients with multiple sclerosis. Frontiers in Neurology. 2022;**13**:931014

[22] Brandle SM, Obermeier B, Senel M, Bruder J, Mentele R, Khademi M, et al. Distinct oligoclonal band antibodies in multiple sclerosis recognize ubiquitous self-proteins. Proceedings of the National Academy of Sciences of the United States of America. 2016;**113**(28):7864-7869

[23] Freedman MS, Thompson EJ, Deisenhammer F, Giovannoni G, Grimsley G, Keir G, et al. Recommended standard of cerebrospinal fluid analysis in the diagnosis of multiple sclerosis: A consensus statement. Archives of Neurology. 2005;**62**(6):865-870

[24] Kuhle J, Kropshofer H, Haering DA, Kundu U, Meinert R, Barro C, et al. Blood neurofilament light chain as a biomarker of MS disease activity and treatment response. Neurology. 2019;**92**(10):e1007-e1015

[25] Khademi M, Kockum I, Andersson ML, Iacobaeus E, Brundin L, Sellebjerg F, et al. Cerebrospinal fluid CXCL13 in multiple sclerosis: A suggestive prognostic marker for the disease course. Multiple Sclerosis. 2011;**17**(3):335-343

[26] Agah E, Zardoui A, Saghazadeh A, Ahmadi M, Tafakhori A, Rezaei N. Osteopontin (OPN) as a CSF and blood biomarker for multiple sclerosis: A systematic review and meta-analysis. PLoS One. 2018;**13**(1):e0190252

[27] Fainardi E, Castellazzi M, Bellini T, Manfrinato MC, Baldi E, Casetta I, et al. Cerebrospinal fluid and serum levels and intrathecal production of active matrix

metalloproteinase-9 (MMP-9) as markers of disease activity in patients with multiple sclerosis. Multiple Sclerosis. 2006;**12**(3):294-301

[28] Huang J, Khademi M, Fugger L, Lindhe O, Novakova L, Axelsson M, et al. Inflammation-related plasma and CSF biomarkers for multiple sclerosis. Proceedings of the National Academy of Sciences of the United States of America. 2020;**117**(23):12952-12960

Section 2

Biomarkers and Genetics in Multiple Sclerosis

Chapter 2

Biomarkers in Multiple Sclerosis

Valentina Ignatova

Abstract

Clinical, biological, and radiological evidence are currently needed to diagnose MS, but lack of preclinical biomarkers hinders the earliest possible diagnosis and treatment. Conventional biomarkers target immunity, blood-brain barrier disruption, demyelination, and neuronal and axonal damage, as well as mitochondrial activity. An increase of specific brain metabolites with 30–40% is registered before detection of MRI lesions in MS. Potential lipid biomarkers are fatty acids, phospholipids, and oxysterols. The role of proteoforms in the pathogenesis of MS was confirmed. Serum neurofilament light chains (sNfL) are currently being studied as a readily available biomarker for prognosis and response to treatment in MS. The sNfL levels reflect ongoing neuroaxonal damage caused by inflammation, and the sNfL levels predict disease activity over the next few years. The retinal nerve fiber layer (RNFL) thinning is reliable as a biomarker of disability worsening. The neutrophil-to-lymphocyte ratio and CRP are also MS biomarkers. The development of rationally targeted therapeutic agents that allow preventive treatment to stop the disease is also delayed without definite biomarkers.

Keywords: biomarkers, multiple sclerosis, diagnostic, progression, monitoring of immunomodulatory therapy, disease activity

1. Introduction

MS is a chronic disease with autoimmune genesis and social significance, which affects the young persons and manifests clinically with unpredictable relapses and subsequent remissions and/or debilitating progression over time [1]. About 2.5 million people worldwide suffer from MS and women are at least 2-3 times more likely to get the illness than men. Other factors identified in the distribution of the disease include genetics, environment, and ethnic origin [2].

Pathophysiologically, a chronic inflammatory reaction occurs in the CNS, leading to multifocal demyelination of axons in white and gray matter. Axon damage also occurs, leading to neuronal loss and atrophy of the brain and spinal cord [2]. Histopathological studies show that reactive astrocytes in freshly developed plaques release chemokines, which activate microglia and increase the permeability of the blood-brain barrier. This in turn allows the migration of macrophages and T lymphocytes into the brain parenchyma [3]. Therefore, astroglial activation may be an important trigger for the cascade of the immune system, leading to neuronal damage, inflammatory demyelination, and axonal degeneration. On the other hand, damaged astrocytes in chronic lesions are involved in the formation of gliotic scars; therefore, astroglia may also be involved in the neurodegeneration process along with axonal damage. In fact, neurodegeneration is the main reason for the accumulation of disability and clinical progression of the disease [4].

Diagnosis of MS is often difficult and is currently based on the 2017 revision of the McDonald's criteria, which include clinical neurological examination, the presence of oligoclonal bands (OCBs) in the cerebrospinal fluid (CSF), magnetic resonance imaging (MRI), and the most accurate possible exclusion of diseases related to the differential diagnosis [5]. The main concept in the diagnosis of MS is the coexistence of clinical and imaging indicators showing both spatial distribution (DIS; involvement of different CNS sites) and temporal distribution (DIT; showing chronic disease, e.g., 2 relapses) [6]. Assessment of cerebral atrophy may also be important if it is measured routinely [7].

The disease is categorized into three main phenotypes: relapsing-remitting MS (RRMS), primary progressive MS (PPMS), and secondary progressive MS (SPMS). Disability and severity of MS are assessed according to the Extended Disability Status Scale (EDSS) [2]. MS shows great heterogeneity in terms of radiological and histopathological findings, clinical course, and progression, as well as in terms of therapeutic response [7, 8]. Therefore, it is very important to identify reliable biomarkers as specific characteristics of the disease that facilitate diagnosis and prognosis and to allow assessment of therapeutic response and risk of side effects [6, 7]. Unfortunately, there is currently no biomarker available to meet the criteria for a surrogate endpoint in MS. It is also clear that biomarkers will play a very important role in MS research and clinical practice in the future.

The purpose of the present work is to analyze the role of the potential biomarkers identified as a result of current research.

2. Definition and nature of biomarkers

The Biomarkers Definitions Working Group gave the following international definition of biomarkers: a characteristic that can be measured objectively and could differentiate the physiological biological phenomena from pathological processes, as well as evaluate the pharmacological reactions to the administered drugs [9]. Biomarker type 0 is considered as a marker for the natural history of the disease and corresponds longitudinally with the known clinical indicators. Biomarker type I perceives the effects of therapeutic procedure including its action mechanism. The surrogate endpoint is a biomarker that is expected as a substitute for a clinically relevant endpoint and serves as a predictor of the therapeutic effect. The clinical endpoint is a clinically relevant measure of how a patient feels, functions, or survives. Evaluation criteria for defining clinical utility of biomarkers include sensitivity/specificity, reliability, evaluation of biomarkers in epidemiological studies or cohorts with natural disease history, evaluation of biomarkers in evidence from clinical trials, evaluation of biomarkers in large multicenter therapeutic studies, evaluation of biomarkers in meta-analyzes, and mathematical modeling of the relationship between a biomarker and a clinical endpoint [10].

The NIH and the FDA have jointly developed a definition for biomarkers, which to be followed both by researchers in their work on obtaining relevant evidence and by practicing specialists to apply biomarkers in healthcare. Different organizations such as Clinical Trials Transformation Initiative and Foundation for National Institutes of Health The Biomarkers Consortium must follow the expansion of this activity. As a result of their joint efforts common definitions have been formulated, which have gained publicity through the constant updating of the online document "Biomarkers, Endpoints, and other Tools" (BEST) [11].

The ideal biomarker should be a binary value or in other words a characteristic that is detected in persons with a specific disease and is not identified in healthy individuals or in subjects with different diseases or vice versa. If the illness progresses or improves, the biomarker's concentration should be increased or decreased, respectively [7, 12]. Establishing the ideal biomarker should be safe for the subject and it should be easily identified, and recommendatory in noninvasive way. Sensitivity and specificity are other key criteria for biomarkers. Sensitivity describes the proportion of truly positive test results among those who are actually affected by the disease. Specificity, on the other hand, shows the proportion of true negative outcomes among those who are not ill. Since high sensitivity is usually due to a lower specificity and opposite, it is important to find biomarkers that reach a satisfactory balance between the two characteristics. Other significant criteria for the biomarkers are their positive and negative predicted value. They show the proportion of correctly/incorrectly diagnosed patients depending on the positive or negative test result. Last but not least is the transfer of biomarkers from research into clinical practice [13].

3. Requirements for MS biomarkers

The classification of MS-specific biomarkers should be based on a careful assessment of all contributing pathophysiological processes. Based on an analysis of published studies investigating the pathophysiological mechanisms of MS Bielekova and Martin classify the majority of proposed biomarkers in MS in one of the following categories: [10].

I. Immunologic biomarkers:

1. Cytokines and cytokine receptors
2. Chemokines and chemokine receptors
3. Antibodies
4. Biomarkers, related to complement system
5. Adhesion molecules
6. Biomarkers reflecting the processing and presentation of antigens
7. Other activation biomarkers
8. Biomarkers associated with cell cycle and apoptosis

II. Markers reflecting immune-associated neuroprotection:

1. Changes in cellular subpopulations
2. Functional tests for immunological reactivity
3. Biomarkers for the state of blood-brain barrier (BBB)

III. Biomarkers for demyelinating lesions

IV. Biomarkers for oxidative stress and excitotoxicity

V. Biomarkers for axonal/neuronal damage

VI. Biomarkers for gliosis

VII. Biomarkers for remyelination and repair

For neurological diseases such as MS, CSF, given its proximity to the CNS, would be the preferred body fluid to look for candidate biomarkers rather than plasma or serum. However, it is clear that CSF sampling is a more invasive procedure with potential risks than plasma sampling. However, the availability of leakage or release of products from different tissues or blood cells in the plasma may correspond with pathological and physiological condition of the specific tissues. Since that plasma is easy to be received in noninvasive way, it can be proposed as a useful fluid for deriving promising diagnostic biomarkers [14].

According to the functional classification provided by the FDA-NIH Biomarker Working Group, molecular biomarkers for MS can be categorized by sensitivity, diagnosis, monitoring, prognosis, safety, and response biomarkers (**Table 1**) [15].

Biomarker	Status	Function	Evidence
IGG OCB	Clinically useful	Diagnostic	Nearly 80% specificity and more than 90% sensitivity for the MS diagnosis. Implemented in 2017 McDonald diagnostic criteria for MS
		Prognostic for conversion	Associated with higher risk for conversion in MS when detected CIS and RIS
IGG index	Clinically useful	Diagnostic	Positive values found in 70–80% of MS patients. Useful as complementary tool, without replacing CSF OCB
		Disease activity	Associated with MRI activity
		Prognostic for conversion	Associated with higher risk of conversion in MS when detected in CIS
		Prognostic for progression	Associated with disease progression
KFLC	Validated	Diagnostic	Useful for MS diagnosis; increased levels detected in MS patients without IGG OCB
		Prognostic for conversion	Associated with higher risk of conversion in MS when detected in CIS
		Prognostic for progression	Associated with disability progression
IGM OCB	Validated	Disease activity	Associated with aggressive disease course
		Prognostic for conversion	Lipid-specific IGM OCB is associated with higher risk of conversion in CIS
		Prognostic for progression	Associated with disability progression and conversion to SPMS
		Treatment response	Lipid-specific IGM OCB predicts a decreased response to IFN beta

Biomarker	Status	Function	Evidence
N-CAM	Validated	Diagnostic	Lower levels detected in MS patients in PPMS compared to RRMS. Indicator of poor remyelination and repair
		Disease activity	Increased levels detected after relapses, especially under steroid treatment, and related to clinical remission
CHI3L1	Validated	Diagnostic	Increased levels in MS and NMO
		Prognostic for conversion	Associated with higher risk of conversion in MS from CIS
		Disease activity	Increased levels in higher clinical and MRI activity
		Treatment response	Increased levels in non-responder patients on INF beta treatment compared to responders
NFs	Validated	Prognostic for conversion	In RIS increased NF-L is independent risk for conversion to CIS and MS, with greater values related to shorter time of conversion
		Disease activity	Double NF-L levels in relapsing patients compared with remitting ones. CSF NF-L levels correlate with NEDA-3, MRI activity, and brain atrophy. Serum NF-L in early phase contributed to predicting the lesion load and brain volume loss over a period of 10 years
		Prognosis for progression	High NF-L is associated with progression in both clinically stable patients and relapsing ones. In CIS patients without ON, CSF NF-L predicts long-term cognitive and physical disability over a period of 9-19 years; higher NF-H

Table 1.
Up-to-date clinically useful and validated MS biomarkers from CSF.

4. Types of biomarkers according to molecular characteristic

4.1 Neurofilaments

Neurofilaments are neuron-specific intermediate filaments formed from etheropolymers of protein subunits with low (neurofilament light [NF-L]) (68 kDa), medium neurofilament medium) (160 kDa) and high (neurofilament heavy [NF-H]) (205 kDa) molecular weight [13]. They are the main components of the cytoskeleton of neurons. Their relative stability and abundance in CNS tissue make them ideal candidates for biomarkers [16]. Levels of neurofilament in biological fluids, particularly CSF, are thought to reflect the degree of axonal damage based on their release into the extracellular space during axonal damage. Neurofilament (NFL) levels are elevated during all stages of MS, especially in relapsing-remitting MS and in progressive MS, while NFL levels decrease to normal during intervention with disease-modifying therapies, suggesting that NFL is associated with various pathological processes involved in MS, reflecting disease activity, disease progression, and treatment efficacy [16]. Interestingly, NF-L and NF-H levels do not always correlate directly with each other, perhaps due to differences in protein stability and sensitivity of the assay. It is thought that NF-L is associated rather with the initial inflammatory stage of MS, as it detects early acute, inflammatory-mediated axonal damage, and correlates weaker with disability progression. On the other hand, NF-H is considered as a marker of neurodegeneration since it highly corresponds with the axonal damage in the course of disease progression [13]. Elevated sNfL levels are prognostic short- and long-term markers, including recurrence, progression of disability, development of MRI lesions, and loss of brain volume [17].

4.2 Chitinase 3-like proteins

Chitinases represent secreted glycoproteins, united in a family, which bind and hydrolyze chitin. Chitinase I (CHIT1) or chitotriosidase, Chitinase 3-like-1 (CHqI3L1), and Chitinase 3-like-2 CHI3L2) are proteins, homologous to chitinases, which bind with chitin, but do not have the capacity to hydrolyze it. In brain tissue in MS, CHI3L1 (also known as YKL-40) and CHI3L2 are expressed in astrocytes in white matter plaques and in normal-looking white matter, and CHI3L1 is also expressed in microglia in MS lesions. Validation in larger cohorts will be required before they can be used as part of the general clinical practice of MS [13].

4.3 Biomarkers of innate immunity

Due to expansion of understanding of the involvement of microglia and macrophages in MS, CNS biomarkers for innate immune activation are needed to be established for evaluation of the course of the disease and efficacy of the immunomodulating therapies. The detection of soluble cell surface biomarkers in CSF could determine the immune phenotype of intrathecal inflammation in MS. Biomarkers derived from the myeloid line such as soluble CD163 (sCD163) and sCD14 are secreted by monocytes and are elevated only in CSF of MS patients. sCD1 correlates weakly with the absolute number of monocytes in CSF, suggesting that the sCD14/monocyte ratio could be used as a marker for activation of microglia. Several studies suggest that sCD163 may be a biomarker of macrophage activity because of its good correlation with monocyte count in CSF of MS persons. Quantification of intrathecal sCD production revealed an increased CSF/serum ratio of sCD163 in persons with RRMS and PPMS, in parallel with other biomarkers of inflammation and neurodegeneration, including elevated NF-L in CSF. The trigger receptor expressed on myeloid cells 2 (TREM-2) is found at high levels in CNS microglia, where it may play a role in weakening the immune response. Soluble TREM-2 increased in CSF in MS patients and decreased after natalizumab treatment [13]. Immunoglobulin (Ig) M and IgG antibodies revealed as OCBs in CSF are considered to reflect the antigen-driven pathophysiology in MS, albeit the certain antigens are still unclear. Intrathecal OCBs, in particular IgG, are a hallmark of MS and are the most commonly applied diagnostic biomarkers in MS, although it is not specific to the disease [13].

Azzolini et al. found a significant positive correlation between IL-9 and TREM-2 CSF levels. In EAE and MS IL-9 is associated with anti-inflammatory action and neuroprotection. IL-9 reduces the activation of macrophages and microglia, inhibits the release of pro-inflammatory molecules, and promotes the anti-inflammatory phenotype [18]. The correlation between GFAP and sTREM-2 and the levels of different inflammatory cytokines is consistent with the cross-link between CSF inflammation and the activation of microglia and astroglia in MS [19].

4.4 Circulating microRNA (miRNAs)

MicroRNA (miRNAs) are a class of small noncoding RNAs consisting of 17–25 nucleotides, whose main role is gene regulation by mediating mRNA degradation, as well as by regulating transcription and translation. miRNAs form up to 1% of the human genome [20]. Circulating miRNAs, usually packaged in microvesicles or exosomes, are relatively stable. They are found in most biofluids, such as CSF, serum, plasma, and whole blood and peripheral blood mononuclear cells (PBMCs). miRNAs are detected through multiple methods such as quantitative PCR, miRNA array analysis, small noncoding RNA cloning, or next-generation sequencing. Dysregulation of miRNAs may play an important role in the underlying mechanisms of MS and potentially serve as a reference for measuring disease progression [13].

4.5 Proteoma

Based on analysis of protein spots of interest seven differentially expressed proteins in CSF samples from RRMS-patients compared to subjects with other inflammatory diseases of the CNS were identified, as determined by 2D-PAGE, respectively Alpha-1-antichymotrypsin, prostaglandin D synthase (PGDS), retinol-binding protein-4 (Rbp4), transthyretin (TTR), apolipoprotein E (ApoE), and gelsolin and angiotensinogen [21]. The most striking change in the CSF proteome in RRMS is the oligomerization of TTR in high molecular weight species (conformers) in about 70% of the analyzed samples. Proteomic studies have shown a decrease in alpha-1-antichymotrypsin in the CSF of patients with RRMS compared with samples collected from patients with other inflammatory diseases of the CNS. This is supported by the results obtained in the validation of studies using ELISA in both sexes [14, 21].

4.6 Metabolomic

Metabolomics is a promising technique that studies small molecules (<1500 Da) in various biological matrices, including cells, biofluids such as serum, plasma, cerebrospinal fluid (CSF), urine, feces, tissues, and exhaled gases. Metabolomics has gained notoriety in recent years for its usefulness in identifying potential biomarkers of MS and providing insight into the pathogenesis of the disease. A growing number of studies show that metabolomics is a promising tool for the diagnosis and prognosis of MS [22].

4.7 Kappa free light chains (KFLC) in CSF

Kappa free light chains (KFLC) in the cerebrospinal fluid (CSF) are promising biomarkers for multiple sclerosis (MS), especially the kappa (K) index.

Martins et al. determine KFLC in CSF and serum samples of patients with MS, clinically/radiologically isolated syndrome (N = 39), and controls (N = 152; inflammatory and noninflammatory neurological diseases). The researchers found higher KFLC parameters in the MS group and the K index performed best among them (AUC 0.92). At a limit of 7.25, it showed better sensitivity (85% vs. 77%) but less specificity (88% vs. 91%) than OCBs. The effectiveness of the IgG index was lower (AUC 0.83). A K index threshold of 2.55 (97% sensitivity) would reduce OCB testing by 52% in the study population. The proposed threshold of 7.25 may help diagnose MS and identify some false-negative cases from OCB studies [23].

4.8 CNS endothelial-derived extracellular vesicles (EEVs)

Mazzucco et al. conducted the first study in which CNS EEVs or EVs derived from BBB were identified in human circulation. The authors develop a new method for identifying EVs derived from CNS endothelial cells by detecting multiple cell-specific markers on EVs isolated from the patient's plasma by flow cytometry. Using this method, the researchers identified three different populations of CNS-EEV including CNS-EEV31, CNS-EEV105, and CNS-EEV144. The scientists found that CNS-EEV concentrations were higher in patients with RRMS with active disease than in HC, stable in patients with RRMS who did not receive disease-modifying therapies (DMT), stable in patients with RRMS who were not receiving natalizumab, and stable in patients with RRMS receiving ocrelizumab [24].

5. Types of biomarkers according to clinical characteristics of MS

5.1 Diagnostic biomarkers for MS

Biomarkers that are suitable for the diagnosis of MS should be able to distinguish MS patients from healthy people or from those with other diseases [7].

A 30–40% increase in specific metabolites (e.g. choline) was detected by proton magnetic resonance spectroscopy in the brain prior to MRI detection of lesions in normal-looking white matter [25]. Decreases in N-acetylaspartate have been found in the brain areas of MS patients and correlated with impairment in which conventional MRI images failed to show a correlation [26, 27]. The results of Ferreira et al. show for the first time that serum phospholipid in MS is significantly different from that of healthy controls and that it may be suitable as biomarkers for clinical applications for MS [27, 28].

CRP is a nonspecific reagent in the acute phase, as it is influenced by several factors, such as infections, inflammation, smoking, and body mass index. DMTs generating lymphopenia can cause higher NLR [29].

Momtazmanesh et al. found significantly higher levels of NFL in the CSF of patients with CIS compared to healthy persons. GFAP levels are remarkably higher in the CSF of MS patients compared to controls. In general, CSF t-tau levels are higher in MS patients with moderate significance. Both CHI3L1 and S100B levels are significantly higher in the CSF of MS patients compared to controls [30].

OCBs were introduced in 1983 as a diagnostic criterion for MS and thus represent the first biomarker of this disease [31, 32]. Since OCBs, meanwhile, have not been used for diagnostics according to McDonald's 2010 criteria, they are again part of the diagnostic algorithm in the 2017 update [33]. CSF IgG OCB is found in almost 90% of patients with MS and in nearly 70% of patients with CIS [34]. Of all the possible models, type 2 is detected when at least two IgG bands are present in the CSF but not in the serum, suggesting intrathecal IgG synthesis and thus inflammatory CNS disease [35].

Immunoglobulin (Ig) G index indicates the ratio of IgG in CSF/serum compared to CSF/serum reference protein albumin. Albumin ratio, i.e., the albumin in CSF/the albumin in serum, is a measure of impaired blood-CSF barrier function in MS. The IgG index is applied as a marker for intrathecal synthesis of immunoglobulins. An IgG index >0.7 is an indicator of an increased intrathecal B-cell response and thus indicates the presence of MS [36]. About 70% of MS patients have an elevated IgG index.

Several studies have reported an increased concentration of free light chains in the CSF of patients with MS [37]. The KFLC index corresponds positively with the IgG index, which is a measure of intrathecal synthesis [38], using a cut-off value of 5. KFLS shows greater sensitivity (more than 96% vs. almost 50% for IgG index) for the detection of OCB (IgG) in CSF and diagnosis of MS and in regard to the negative prognosis it has comparable specificity. According to consensus report from 1994 on the role of CSF in MS diagnosis, the intrathecal Ig-synthesis against viruses, such as measles, rubella, and varicella zoster, is used as a complementary diagnostic exam in MS [39]. Such kind of local humoral response, known as measles-rubella-varicella-zoster (MRZ) response (MRZR), is registered in about 94% of persons with MS in case of at least one intrathecal virus-specific response is found, and the anti-measles response is the most common [40].

5.2 Biomarkers for MS-progression

5.2.1 Biomarkers for conversion from CIS to MS

Neuronal and glial biomarkers may be useful in determining the risk of conversion to MS in patients with CIS or RIS [31]. In patients with RIS, elevated CSF levels NF-L > 619 ng/L have been shown to be an independent risk factor for conversion to CIS and MS [41]. CHI3L1 levels in CSF correlate with the time of conversion from CIS to MS. However, the correlation did not remain significant for patients when followed for more than 5 years [42]. Other studies with a follow-up period of less than 3 years found that CHI3L1 levels in CSF were not a predictor of conversion in patients with CIS. No correlation was found between the baseline levels of the other markers (t-tau, GFAP, and S100B) and the conversion time from CIS to MS [42].

The results from actual research show that detection of CSF OCB in children with RIS is associated with increased risk of developing pediatric MS and also improves the specificity of MRI criteria in this population [43]. Another study on 75 RIS patients confirmed that CSF OCB was an independent risk factor for conversion from RIS to CIS and to MS, which happened for a shorter time [44]. In patients with CIS, the identification of CSF lipid-specific IgM OCB is associated with an increased MRI lesion load and brain atrophy at the first clinical event with an aggressive course of the disease. The load on periventricular lesions in the first years of the disease is also associated with the formation of intrathecal IgM synthesis in patients with CIS, so it is assumed that IgM plays an active role in the development of demyelinating lesions [45]. In another study by Ferraro et al., the identification of CSF IgM OCB in patients with CIS predicted another recurrence within 1 year [46]. The results of a blinded multicenter study involving 52 neurological patients and 13 centers confirmed the reproducibility of the test [47]. OCBs in CIS patients also predict a more aggressive course of the disease and correlate with brain atrophy, lesion load, and elevated CSF levels of CXCL13, a chemokine that directs B cell migration [13].

In a study by Comabella and colleagues, CSF CHI3L1 levels were further correlated with shorter latency conversion times and with the progression of disability during follow-up and radiological activity of the disease [48]. High levels of glial markers for activation of YKL-40 and GFAP are associated with earlier progression to EDSS 3 and that high levels of YKL-40 are also associated with earlier progression to EDSS 6. Martínez et al. also reported higher levels of YKL-40 in patients with CIS with a reduced time to conversion to CDMS, which supports the results of a previous study [49]. However, the prognostic value of YKL-40 is lost when the conversion time is extended by more than 5 years. These findings further suggest that glial activation may play a key role in the progression of MS [13, 42].

5.2.2 Markers of disease progression

GFAP and sTREM-2 have been studied in MS as useful tools for monitoring disease progression. Serum and CSF concentrations of GFAP have also been associated with clinical impairment and radiological activity [50]. In patients with progressive MS, serum GFAP concentrations are related to age and EDSS, as well as to neurofilament light levels (NF-L) [19, 51]. Increased expression of pro-inflammatory molecules, including IL-1β, IL-2, IL-6, and IL-8, has been associated with higher disease prospective activity, impairment, and neurodegeneration in MS [52, 53].

Guzel et al. [54] found that both CRP and NLR had discriminatory capacity for patients with EDSS > 5 versus EDSS ≤5.36. Demirci et al. [55] concluded that NLR may be a potential predictor of disability progression, and Bisgaard et al. categorizes NLR as an additional marker [56]. No significant difference was found between NFL CSF levels in RRMS (N = 752) compared to PMS (N = 462) patients based on a meta-analysis summarizing several studies [31].

In a study of 29 MS patients who were followed for 5–16 years, the presence of CSF IgM OCB was strongly associated with conversion to SPMS and achieving a higher EDSS score [57, 58]. In other studies, serum GFAP levels were also associated with higher EDSS scores but also with longer disease duration and progressive course [42, 59]. Earlier studies have also found associations between miRNAs expression and MS damage or disease progression.

Higher NfL are associated with a higher subsequent rate of whole-brain atrophy, and recent inflammatory activity (new/increasing T2 lesions), as well as T2LV, is associated with higher NfL [60]. Clinically significant prognostic value of NF-H was also recently demonstrated in a cohort of 51 patients followed for an average of 15 years [13, 17].

Regarding the diagnosis of primary progressive MS (PPMS), the presence of CSF OCB is one of the mandatory criteria [33] and its role has been confirmed over time in successive revisions following the Poser criteria [61].

5.3 Biomarkers as indicators for the efficacy of the DMT

The therapeutic benefit of some DMTs, such as interferon beta (IFNβ) and natalizumab, often weakens due to neutralizing antibodies production. These serum antibodies are routinely tested during certain periods and are used as biomarkers for the effect of treatment. The myxovirus resistance protein (MxA) is another valuable biomarker of the IFNβ response frequently used in clinical practice.

CSF NF-L was reduced in patients after switching from IFN or glatiramer acetate to rituximab, which correlates with traditional NMR measurements for inflammatory activity, further supporting CSF NF-L as a measure of disease activity. NfL has shown utility as a biomarker for treatment with fingolimod, siponimod, natalizumab, and ocrelizumab in PMS cohorts [13].

Natalizumab has been associated with progressive multifocal leukoencephalopathy (PML) caused by reactivation of the JC virus in the CNS. The risk of PML is monitored by prospective serum testing of JCV antibodies. Currently, the use of a "PML risk stratification test" that measures the level of anti-JCV antibodies through an ELISA-based test in patients receiving natalizumab is helpful. Altered levels of miRNAs in PBMCs are normalized by autologous hematopoietic stem cell transplantation and natalizumab. Regarding the risks of natalizumab, several miRNAs are possible biomarkers for the development of PML in patients receiving natalizumab. Fingolimod treatment decreased miR 150 plasma levels and did not affect cerebrospinal fluid (CSF) levels, while natalizumab treatment increased miR-150 plasma levels and decreased CSF levels [13].

NF-L concentrations in CSF have been shown to reduce during the second year of the immunosuppressive therapy in patients with active progressive MS and after switching from first-line therapies to fingolimod in those with RRMS. In addition, CSF NF-L has shown the advantage of better therapeutic biomarker after 12 months of NTZ treatment in subjects with RRMS, compared to NF-H, [62]. However, the potential role of CSF NF-L as a biomarker for response to treatment is severely limited by the invasiveness of performing serial lumbar punctures. Conversely, serial NF-L serum scores would be an easier-to-detect marker and a reliable indicator of NF-L CSF levels [63]. The serum levels of NF-L correlated positively with clinical and radiological activity in MS at baseline and during follow-up, trend to decrease at the 6 months of IMD administration and reached stable values below 8 pg/ml in those subjects who maintained NEDA-3. In addition, persons who expressed clinical and radiological activity of the disease during observation period also showed elevated serum NF-L levels up to 5 months before relapses.

There is not sufficient evidence of possible interactions between DMD and CSF IgM OCB. Patients with RRMS on treatment with IFN-β showed reduced therapeutic response depending on CSF lipid-specific IgM OCB, who experienced a mild reduction of the relapse rate and increased likelihood of reaching deteriorated EDSS. NTZ has been shown to decrease serum IgM and IgG concentrations after 2 years of treatment onset in a time-dependent way [64].

Some studies have examined variations in matrix metalloproteinase (MMP) levels in patients with DMD. Significant reductions in serum MMP-9 mRNA in patients with RRMS below IFN-β have been observed after 12 months of follow-up by Galboiz and colleagues [65] and confirmed by other studies [66]. It is worth noting that a significant elevation of TIMP-1 levels was observed in the group of respondents compared to nonrespondents [67]. A possible therapeutic effect to NTZ treatment has also been studied. Balasa and colleagues found a significant reduction of MMP-9 in the serum after 8 months of treatment onset and a positive correlation between the biomarker concentration and the disease activity [68], but this finding has not been affirmed by other research [69]. Decreased baseline MMP-9 levels were found in patients treated with NTZ in patients who developed progressive multifocal leukoencephalopathy compared to those who did not [70].

In patients with CIS, in parallel with the assessment of the risk of conversion, it is important to choose the adequate treatment decisions preferably supported by biomarkers that could predict the future course of the disease. For example, biomarkers associated with axonal damage or oligodendroglial waste could facilitate the recognition of subjects who need aggressive and early treatment approaches to suppress the disease progression and long-term disability [13].

5.4 Markers of MS activity

CRP and NLR as biomarkers of disease activity in MS. NLRs appear to reflect better systemic inflammation than specific neutrophil and lymphocyte counts alone. NLR is calculated as the ratio of the number of neutrophils to lymphocytes, which makes it a simple, fast, nonspecific, and inexpensive way to detect increased systemic inflammation. NLR as a biomarker comes from observations showing that systemic inflammation regularly leads to neutrophilia and lymphocytopenia [29].

Nitric oxide metabolites. Due to the role of oxidative stress in the pathogenesis of MS, nitrates and nitrites have been studied as biomarkers of disease activity [71].

Interferon-beta (IFN-β) has shown remarkable inhibition of inducible expression of NO synthase in astrocytes [72–74]. Significantly higher levels of nitrites and nitrates were found in patients with relapse than in remission and patients treated with steroids in the previous 1–2 months [74, 75]. Accordingly, NO metabolites predict disease activity with 71% specificity and 66% susceptibility [76].

Osteopontin. Osteopontin (OPN) is closely linked to the immune system. In its soluble form, it is secreted by macrophages and activated leukocytes and also interacts with them, reducing the inducible form of NO synthase, and stimulating inflammatory process. In its intracellular form, OPN is expressed by dendritic cells and promotes the differentiation of Th17 and Treg [77]. OPN is probably facilitating increased regulation of Th1 and Th17 cytokines, mostly IFN-γ and IL-17 [78, 79]. A specific subset of Th1 cells, particularly those occurring in CSF during relapses, are thought to produce OPN, high levels of IFN-γ, and matrix metalloproteinase-9 (MMP-9) after polyclonal stimulation, playing a pathogenetic role [80, 81].

C-X-C motif ligand 13. The C-X-C motif ligand 13 (CXCL13), also known as a chemokine that attracts B cells (BCA-1), is a protein that promotes the chemotaxis of mature B lymphocytes by interacting with its CXCR5 receptor [79]. In fact, CXCL13 has been found to be overexpressed in active MS lesions and in intrameningeal B-cell follicles of chronic white matter lesions, maintaining humoral autoimmunity and disease activity [82, 83]. In a study by Khademi et al. CSF CXCL13 was found to be significantly higher in infectious neurological diseases and MS [84].

MMP-9. During inflammation, many molecules are able to activate MMPs, including reactive oxygen species and TNF-α and IL-17 via NF-κB [85]. It has been suggested that MMPs may also act in MS by digesting myelin basic protein (MBP), in addition to promoting leukocyte leakage into postcapillary venules [86].

Myelin basic protein. It has long been known that MBP is a potential biomarker of disease activity for MS, as it shows acute CNS myelin damage, although it is not disease-specific. Several studies have found elevated levels of MBP in CSF in MS patients temporarily associated with relapses [87] and detectable up to 5–6 weeks later [88]. Accordingly, patients with RRMS with disease activity showed higher values than progressive MS and stable patients [89]. MBP concentrations in CSF are also higher when polysymptomatic and severe relapses occur, which correlates with EDSS score and MRI activity and decreases after treatment with corticosteroids [90].

Neuronal cell adhesion molecule (N-CAM). The adhesion molecule of neuronal cells (N-CAM) is considered a marker for recovery and remyelination and is expressed mainly in the CNS [91].

5.5 Biomarkers for MS relapses

Patients with recurrent MS have higher levels of CSF NFL than patients in remission. No significant difference in GFAP CSF levels was found between patients in relapse and remission. The difference in CSF t-tau levels between patients with relapse and remission was not significant [30].

The results of Martínez et al. are consistent with previous studies showing higher NFL levels during relapse [30, 41]. The authors confirm the conclusion of a previous study by Malmeström et al. that NFL levels decrease further 60 days after the onset of relapse [92]. Conversely, MCP-1 levels increase in the stable phases of the disease, indicating that this marker may reflect an anti-inflammatory effect [93].

In a group of patients with active recurrent and progressive MS, Thebault et al. showed that increased sNfL at baseline and also longitudinal elevation of sNfL from previously low baseline values predict relapse manifestations over a 12-month follow-up period. Increased baseline sNfL rates are also corresponding with subsequent gadolinium-enhanced lesions during disease activity and with deterioration of disability. sGFAP is associated with upcoming MRI activity only, but not with other parameters [17].

In patients with milder relapses, treated with drugs on first-line, the sNfL levels are more stable than in severe relapsed subjects. In MS patients with more active course of the disease, increased sNfL was observed 5 months before appearance of new crisis and almost 80% of the increased sNfL (>3 SD) were corresponding with clinical and MRI activity of the disease. Although these group-level observations are important evidence that dynamic change in sNfL is appropriate, utility at the individual patient level is limited [17].

The results of Martínez, 2015 are consistent with previous studies showing higher levels of NFL during relapse [41]. Researchers confirm previous findings that NFL decreases further after 60 days of relapse [92]. This model has not been observed for other biomarkers.

5.6 Biomarkers for neuronal and glial damage in the differentiation of MS subtypes

GFAP alone has been shown to be a useful biomarker for differentiating different MS subtypes. Patients with PMS had higher GFAP levels than RRMS. No significant difference in S100B CSF levels was found between patients with RRMS and SPMS [30]. While in RRMS the movement of adaptive immune cells from the periphery to the CNS is the main pathological mechanism, in PMS the players of innate immunity, including astrocytes and microglia, play a more important role. Molecular biomarkers of reactive astrogliosis show promising results in the differentiation of RRMS and PMS. This may be one of the reasons for the higher levels of GFAP, which reflect astrogliosis, in patients with PMS compared to RRMS. Serum GFAP levels are also higher in patients with SPMS compared to RRMS.

No significant difference was found between t-tau levels in CSF in RRMS compared to PMS. No significant difference was found between the CSF levels of CHI3L1 in RRMS compared to PMS [30]. Metabolic serum metabolic profiling may reveal reliable biomarkers for distinguishing between RRMS, SPMS, and PPMS.10. Metabolic profiling of CSF is currently being developed, but all of these studies require further validation before clinical use [13].

5.7 Association of biomarkers for neuronal and glial disorders with age and sex

Recent meta-analysis has shown that CSF NFL levels are positively correlated with age in HC, but they do not have or have a negative correlation with age in MS. Abnormal changes during the course of MS affecting CSF NFL levels are considered as main feature, differentiating MS patients form HC [30].

A meta-regression analysis showed a negative correlation between the percentage of women and the magnitude of the effect of comparing CSF NFL levels among MS patients. Gender may be a determinant of the CSF levels of neuronal and glial biomarkers of damage. Higher CSF levels of CHI3L1 and t-tau have been found in men suffering from MS. A recent meta-analysis found higher levels of CSF NFL in men in the HC and MS groups. However, in patients with PMS, CSF NFL levels are moderately higher in women. Finally, in addition to CSF levels of biomarkers for neuronal and glial damage, their blood level may also be a practical biomarker in MS. CSF and blood levels of these biomarkers may be affected by DMT and they can potentially be used to monitor the response to treatment.

To date, only GFAP has shown a significant correlation with age, with higher levels found in the elderly [42].

5.8 Biomarkers for cognitive impairment in MS

Cognitive impairment (CI) is a common and disabling symptom in MS. Axonal damage may contribute to the development of CI in the early stages. However, there are currently no biomarkers available to monitor CI in MS patients. Virgilio E et al. in their study aimed to investigate the correlation of axonal biomarkers of CSF, in particular: light chain neurofilaments (NFL), Tau, and beta-amyloid protein (Abeta) in patients with MS with CI at diagnosis. The researchers included 62 newly diagnosed patients with MS and cognition was assessed using the BICAMS battery. CSF levels of NFL, Abeta, and Tau were determined by ELISA. No differences were found in demographic, clinical, and MRI characteristics (with exception of the lower educational level) in persons with CI.

The patients with CI, who accounted for 45.1%, did not differ in demographic, clinical, and MRI parameters (with exception of lower educational level), but showed more severe neurodegeneration, based on higher mean CSF Tau protein (162.1 ± 52.96 pg/ml vs. 132.2 ± 63 pg/ml p: 0.03). No significant differences were reported for Abeta and NFL. A correlation between the number of impaired tests and Tau levels was significant (r: 0.32 p: 0.01). Tau is increased, especially in persons with delayed data rate (IPS) (p: 0.006) and linear regression analysis, subtyping EDSS, MRI, and MS, confirms Tau as a weak predictor of IPS and cognitive impairment. CI has significant impact on the quality of life of MS persons and should be sought even at diagnosis. Biomarkers of axonal damage, in particular Tau, appear to reflect cognitive impairment at the early stages of the disease [94].

In a longitudinal trial on 22 IFNβ-1a- and riluzole-treated patients and 20 IFNβ-1a- and placebo-treated persons with MS at an early stage, the serum NF-L concentrations were evaluated over a 24-month period. The NF-L levels correlated positively with EDSS deterioration, Gd + lesions, and cerebral atrophy. In addition, elevated serum NF-L levels correlated with poorer results in neuropsychological tests that evaluated visual-spatial orientation, recollection, and verbal and nonverbal episodic learning [95]. Similar results on the relationship between serum NF-L levels and CI at the early stages of MS associated with increasing EDSS have been confirmed by other studies. Although the serum NF-L levels correlated with EDSS in patients with PMS, they failed to correspond with EDSS deterioration in the previous year and during a mean follow-up of 27 months. In particular, serum NF-L was elevated in all of the patients with PMS, including those who did not show increasing in EDSS or deepening of the disability [96].

6. Discussion

Many systematic biological approaches such as genomics, epigenomics, and proteomics have been used to expand the knowledge in MS, helping to extract valuable information on the pathogenesis of the disease. Despite this progress, there remains a need for additional tools to understand the exact etiopathogenesis of MS.

There is also a significant unmet need for diagnostic and prognostic biomarkers in MS, especially in progressive forms of the disease [22].

In MS, the potential biomarkers are classified on the basis of their ability to establish the diagnosis, predict the outcomes, and assess the response to treatment. Essentially, the biomarkers for MS need to be able to identify individuals who are vulnerable for receptivity to the disease or at high risk of severe attacks in case of confirmed diagnosis and to predict which individuals are likely to respond to certain treatments. Based on these considerations, many published candidate biomarkers have emerged, although most of them are correlative and have yet to be shown to have significant prognostic potential for the disease. In addition, some biomarkers are common markers of inflammation and, therefore, have no specificity for MS. Nevertheless, they have been shown to be important in elucidating the mechanism of disease, progression, and susceptibility, despite their inability to become practical clinical biomarkers [6].

CSF is a unique source of potential biomarkers for MS, although it requires some invasiveness to collect them. Currently, only diagnostic biomarkers for CSF are used in clinical practice, although hundreds of molecules have been validated as indicating disease activity and prognostic biomarkers. IgG OCBs maintain an important role as a validated diagnostic biomarker and are considered an alternative MRI tool that can replace the spread over time based on the 2017 revision of the McDonald's criteria. They also have a predictive role for conversion from CIS to MS when found in patients with first demyelinating event. NF-L has been shown to be a valuable biomarker that indicates disease activity in MS. The ability to measure NF-L in the serum at different time points makes it suitable for monitoring the response to treatment. The KFLC index was established as a more sensitive but less specific diagnostic biomarker than IgG OCB. It is a potential first-line assessment in patients with suspected MS and minimizes the need for IgG OCB analysis. The KFLC index is a prognostic biomarker for CIS conversion, but the lack of a universal threshold is still a limitation. IgM OCBs have a good potential as a predictive biomarker because of their association with aggressive course of the disease, a higher risk of conversion from CIS to MS, progression of disability, and conversion from RRMS to SPMS. Several biomarkers of the disease activity appear promising, although they require additional validation. Elevated levels of NO metabolites, OPN, MBP, MMP-9, N-CAM, CXCL13, and CHI3L1 were found to be closely correlated with relapses [30, 41]. The role of biomarkers in monitoring the effect of applied BMI is extremely valuable.

Based on the review presented, we can conclude that there are several biomarkers with a degree of relevance in the clinical environment. However, no biomarker is effective in determining diagnosis and prognosis and in terms of sensitivity and specificity. MRI and OCB are currently important in the diagnosis of MS. However, recent studies have shown that the MRZ or NfL reaction is already or may be useful in the future, respectively [6, 32].

The development of biomarkers is comparable to the development of drugs, and independent validation must be demonstrated in large cohorts after a positive pilot test. If biomarker tests are to be used to stimulate patient care, understanding and carefully evaluating these concepts is essential, as "a bad biomarker test is as bad as a bad medicine" [97]. The validation process is often lengthy and usually takes between 5 and 15 years [98]. For this reason, the enrichment of the repertoire of biomarkers for MS has been slow so far.

Biomarkers currently used in clinical practice to diagnose MS include glycoproteins, chemokines, IgG and IgM antibodies, and cellular surface markers of inflammation.

As a step toward a better understanding of the mechanisms of neurodegeneration in MS, recent studies have found new correlations between neurofilaments and other biomarkers of disease activity. CSF NF-L was found to be inversely related to serum vitamin D levels in a group of 153 MS patients [26]. This study suggests that normal or high normal vitamin D levels are not only associated with reduced inflammatory activity in MS but can also protect against axonal damage. It has also been found that axonal damage, measured by neurofilaments, correlates with mitochondrial dysfunction (CSF lactate) and CNS autoimmunity and inhibition of remyelination (CSF lipocalin 2), thus potentially expanding the repertoire of CSF current marker biomarkers. Activity in MS [13].

However, the course of MS disease is very variable and the diversity in the phenotype of the disease is not well related to these biomarkers. Thus, it is imperative to identify new specific biomarkers that can help differentiate clinical phenotypes of MS, predict disease progression, and provide correlation with disability [2].

In addition, biomarkers are needed that reflect the ongoing neurodegeneration, demyelination, and remyelination of gray and white matter, microgliosis, astrogliosis, and oxidative stress, which contribute to the overall activity of the disease. The need is particularly important for progressive MS (SPMS and PPMS), where biomarkers are lacking that can objectively assess the mechanisms of the disease that contribute to neurological deterioration.

Future research is needed to further investigate the clinical use of neuronal and glial biomarkers in MS. More studies are indispensable to shed light on the importance of these markers in differentiating between different phenotypes of MS and the specific course of the disease. Establishing cut-off values for different biomarkers in diagnosing MS and determining its prognosis can be useful [30].

7. Conclusion

Biomarkers are crucial for the emergence of scientific discoveries, for the development of adequate pharmacological products and for quality healthcare for the individual and the population as a whole. The emergence of accurate and reliable biomarkers of CSF, along with the development of safe and effective intrathecal therapies, will make CSF analysis a routine part of optimal clinical management of MS. Peripheral blood collections are less invasive and easier to obtain than CSF collections. Blood biomarkers capable of detecting disease activity in MS and distinguishing different disease phenotypes may be useful in personalized treatment of MS with disease-modifying drugs and predict treatment response. An approach to the development of a biomarker that includes a common regulatory science across multiple disciplines is needed to ensure that evidence-based rational development of biomarkers maintains a pace with scientific and clinical needs.

Conflict of interest

No.

Notes/Thanks/Other declarations

NA.

DOI: http://dx.doi.org/10.5772/intechopen.106052

Author details

Valentina Ignatova
Clinic of Neurology, National Cardiology Hospital, Sofia, Bulgaria

*Address all correspondence to: valyaig@abv.bg

References

[1] Barkhof F, Calabresi PA, Miller DH, et al. Imaging outcomes for neuroprotection and repair in multiple sclerosis trials. Nature Reviews. Neurology. 2009;**5**:256-266

[2] Martinez B, Peplow PV. MicroRNAs in blood and cerebrospinal fluid as diagnostic biomarkers of multiple sclerosis and to monitor disease progression. Neural Regeneration Research. 2020;**15**(4):606

[3] Czeh M, Gressens P, Kaindl AM. The yin and yang of microglia. Developmental Neuroscience. 2011;**33**:199-209

[4] Lassmann H, Brück W, Lucchinetti CF. The immunopathology of multiple sclerosis: An overview. Brain Pathology. 2007;**17**:210-218

[5] McNicholas N, Hutchinson M, McGuigan C, et al. 2017 McDonald diagnostic criteria: A review of the evidence. Multiple Sclerosis and Related Disorders. 2018;**24**:48-54

[6] Arneth B, Kraus J. Laboratory biomarkers of multiple sclerosis (MS). Clinical Biochemistry. 2022;**99**:1-8

[7] Ziemssen T, Akgün K, Brück W. Molecular biomarkers in multiple sclerosis. Journal of Neuroinflammation. 2019;**16**(1):1-11

[8] Inojosa H, Schriefer D, Ziemssen T. Clinical outcome measures in multiple sclerosis: A review. Autoimmunity Reviews. 2020;**19**(5):102512

[9] Biomarkers Definitions Working Group (National Institutes of Health). Biomarkers and surrogate endpoints: Preferred definitions and conceptual framework. Clinical Pharmacology and Therapeutics. 2001;**69**:89-95

[10] Bielekova B, Martin R. Development of biomarkers in multiple sclerosis. Brain. 2004;**127**(7):1463-1478

[11] Califf RM. Biomarker definitions and their applications. Experimental Biology and Medicine. 2018;**243**(3):213-221

[12] Comabella M, Montalban X. Body fluid biomarkers in multiple sclerosis. Lancet Neurology. 2014;**13**:113-126

[13] Harris VK, Tuddenham JF, Sadiq SA. Biomarkers of multiple sclerosis: Current findings. Degenerative Neurological and Neuromuscular Disease. 2017;**7**:19

[14] Nova A, Fazia T, Beecham A, Saddi V, et al. Plasma protein levels analysis in multiple sclerosis Sardinian families identified C9 and CYP24A1 as candidate biomarkers. Life. 2022;**12**(2):151

[15] FDA-NIH Biomarker Working Group. BEST (Biomarkers, EndpointS, and other Tools) Resource [Internet]. Available from: https://www.ncbi.nlm.nih.gov/books/NBK338448/. [Accessed: July 02, 2020]

[16] Cai L, Huang J. Neurofilament light chain as a biological marker for multiple sclerosis: A meta-analysis study. Neuropsychiatric Disease and Treatment. 2018;**14**:2241-2254

[17] Thebault S, Reaume M, Marrie RA, et al. High or increasing serum NfL is predictive of impending multiple sclerosis relapses. Multiple Sclerosis and Related Disorders. 2022;**103535**

[18] Donninelli G, Saraf-Sinik I, Mazziotti V, et al. Interleukin-9 regulates

macrophage activation in the progressive multiple sclerosis brain. Journal of Neuroinflammation. 2020;**17**:149

[19] Azzolini F, Gilio L, Pavone L, et al. Neuroinflammation is associated with GFAP and sTREM2 levels in multiple sclerosis. Biomolecules. 2022;**12**(2):222

[20] Condrat CE, Thompson DC, Barbu MG, et al. miRNAs as biomarkers in disease: Latest findings regarding their role in diagnosis and prognosis. Cell. 2020;**9**(2):276

[21] Salazar IL, Lourenço AS, Manadas B, et al. Posttranslational modifications of proteins are key features in the identification of CSF biomarkers of multiple sclerosis. Journal of Neuroinflammation. 2022;**19**(1):1-23

[22] Liu Z et al. Metabolomics as a promising tool for improving understanding of multiple sclerosis: A review of recent advances. Biomedical Journal. DOI: 10.1016/j.bj.2022.01.004

[23] Martins DA, Lopes J, da Silva A, et al. Kappa free light chains: Diagnostic performance in multiple sclerosis and utility in a clinical laboratory. Clinica Chimica Acta. 2022;**528**:56-64

[24] Mazzucco M, Mannheim W, Shetty S, et al. CNS endothelial derived extracellular vesicles are biomarkers of active disease in multiple sclerosis. Fluids and Barriers of the CNS. 2022;**19**(1):1-24

[25] Narayana PA, Doyle TJ, Lai D, et al. Serial proton magnetic resonance spectroscopic imaging, contrast-enhanced magnetic resonance imaging, and quantitative lesion volumetry in multiple sclerosis. Annals of Neurology. 1998;**43**:56-71

[26] Tur C, Moccia M, Barkhof F, et al. Assessing treatment outcomes in multiple sclerosis trials and in the clinical setting. Nature Reviews. Neurology. 2018;**14**:75

[27] Sen MK, Almuslehi MS, Shortland PJ, et al. Proteomics of multiple sclerosis: Inherent issues in defining the pathoetiology and identifying (early) biomarkers. International Journal of Molecular Sciences. 2021;**22**(14):7377

[28] Ferreira HB, Melo T, Monteiro A, et al. Serum phospholipidomics reveals altered lipid profile and promising biomarkers in multiple sclerosis. Archives of Biochemistry and Biophysics. 2021;**697**:108672

[29] Olsson A, Gustavsen S, Gisselø Lauridsen K, et al. Neutrophil-to-lymphocyte ratio and CRP as biomarkers in multiple sclerosis: A systematic review. Acta Neurologica Scandinavica. 2021;**143**(6):577-586

[30] Momtazmanesh S, Shobeiri P, Saghazadeh A, et al. Neuronal and glial CSF biomarkers in multiple sclerosis: A systematic review and meta-analysis. Reviews in the Neurosciences. 2021;**32**(6):573-595

[31] Poser CM, Paty DW, Scheinberg L, Nald IW, Davis FA, Ebers GC, et al. New diagnostic criteria for multiple sclerosis: Guidelines for research protocols. Annals of Neurology. 1983;**13**:227-231

[32] Ziemssen T, Ziemssen F. The role of the humoral immune system in multiple sclerosis (MS) and its animal model experimental autoimmune encephalomyelitis (EAE). Autoimmunity Reviews. 2005;**4**:460-467

[33] Thompson AJ, Banwell BL, Barkhof F, et al. Diagnosis of multiple sclerosis: 2017 revisions

of the McDonald criteria. Lancet Neurology;2018;**17**(2):162-173

[34] Dobson R, Ramagopalan S, Davis A, et al. Cerebrospinal fluid oligoclonal bands in multiple sclerosis and clinically isolated syndromes: A meta-analysis of prevalence, prognosis and effect of latitude. Journal of Neurology, Neurosurgery, and Psychiatry. 2013;**84**:909-914

[35] Freedman MS, Thompson EJ, Deisenhammer F, et al. Recommended standard of cerebrospinal fluid analysis in the diagnosis of multiple sclerosis: A consensus statement. Archives of Neurology. 2005;**62**:865-870

[36] Maggi P, Absinta M, Grammatico M, et al. Central vein sign differentiates multiple sclerosis from central nervous system inflammatory vasculopathies. Annals of Neurology. 2018;**83**:283-294

[37] Hassan-Smith G, Durant L, Tsentemeidou A, et al. High sensitivity and specificity of elevated cerebrospinal fluid kappa free light chains in suspected multiple sclerosis. Journal of Neuroimmunology. 2014;**276**:175-179

[38] Crespi I, Vecchio D, Serino R, et al. K index is a reliable marker of intrathecal synthesis, and an alternative to IgG index in multiple sclerosis diagnostic work-up. Journal of Clinical Medicine. 2019;**8**:446

[39] Andersson M, Alvarez-Cermeño J, Bernardi G, et al. Cerebrospinal fluid in the diagnosis of multiple sclerosis: A consensus report. Journal of Neurology, Neurosurgery, and Psychiatry. 1994;**57**:897-902

[40] Brettschneider J, Tumani H, Kiechle U, et al. IgG antibodies against measles, rubella, and varicella zoster virus predict conversion to multiple sclerosis in clinically isolated syndrome. PLoS One. 2009;**4**:e7638

[41] Teunissen CE, Iacobaeus E, Khademi M, et al. Combination of N-acetylaspartate and neurofilaments in multiple sclerosis. Neurology. 2009;**72**:1322-1329

[42] Martínez MAM, Olsson B, Bau L, et al. Glial and neuronal markers in cerebrospinal fluid predict progression in multiple sclerosis. Multiple Sclerosis Journal. 2015;**21**(5):550-561

[43] Makhani N, Lebrun C, Siva A, et al. Oligoclonal bands increase the specificity of MRI criteria to predict multiple sclerosis in children with radiologically isolated syndrome. Multiple Sclerosis Journal—Experimental, Translational and Clinical. 2019;**5**:2055217319836664

[44] Matute-Blanch C, Villar LM, Álvarez-Cermeño JC, et al. Neurofilament light chain and oligoclonal bands are prognostic biomarkers in radiologically isolated syndrome. Brain. 2018;**141**:1085-1093

[45] Boscá I, Magraner MJ, Coret F, et al. The risk of relapse after a clinically isolated syndrome is related to the pattern of oligoclonal bands. Journal of Neuroimmunology. 2010;**226**:143-146

[46] Ferraro D, Simone AM, Bedin R, et al. Cerebrospinal fluid oligoclonal IgM bands predict early conversion to clinically definite multiple sclerosis in patients with clinically isolated syndrome. Journal of Neuroimmunology. 2013;**257**:76-81

[47] Espiño M, Abraira V, Arroyo R, et al. Assessment of the reproducibility of oligoclonal IgM band detection for its application in daily clinical practice. Clinica Chimica Acta. 2015;**438**:67-69

[48] Cantó E, Tintoré M, Villar LM, et al. Chitinase 3-like 1: Prognostic biomarker

in clinically isolated syndromes. Brain. 2015;**138**:918-931

[49] Comabella M, Fernández M, Martin R, et al. Cerebrospinal fluid chitinase 3-like 1 levels are associated with conversion to multiple sclerosis. Brain. 2010;**133**:1082-1093

[50] Kassubek R, Gorges M, Schocke M, et al. GFAP in early multiple sclerosis: A biomarker for inflammation. Neuroscience Letters. 2017;**657**:166-170

[51] Abdelhak A, Hottenrott T, Morenas-Rodríguez E, et al. Glial activation markers in CSF and serum from patients with primary progressive multiple sclerosis: Potential of serum GFAP as disease severity marker? Frontiers in Neurology. 2019;**10**:1-9

[52] Rossi S, Studer V, Motta C, et al. Neuroinflammation drives anxiety and depression in relapsing-remitting multiple sclerosis. Neurology. 2017;**89**:1338-1347

[53] Stampanoni Bassi M, Iezzi E, Landi D, et al. Delayed treatment of MS is associated with high CSF levels of IL-6 and IL-8 and worse future disease course. Journal of Neurology. 2018;**265**:2540-2547

[54] Guzel I, Mungan S, Oztekin ZN, et al. Is there an association between the expanded disability status scale and inflammatory markers in multiple sclerosis? Journal of the Chinese Medical Association. 2016;**79**(2):54-57

[55] Demirci S, Demirci S, Kutluhan S, et al. The clinical significance of the neutrophil-to-lymphocyte ratio in multiple sclerosis. International Journal of Neuroscience. 2016;**126**(8):700-706

[56] Bisgaard AK, Pihl-Jensen G, Frederiksen JL. The neutrophil-to-lymphocyte ratio as disease actvity marker in multiple sclerosis and optic neuritis. Multiple Sclerosis and Related Disorders. 2017;**18**:213-217

[57] Villar LM, Masjuan J, González-Porqué P, et al. Intrathecal IgM synthesis is a prognostic factor in multiple sclerosis. Annals of Neurology. 2003;**53**:222-226

[58] Mandrioli J, Sola P, Bedin R, et al. A multifactorial prognostic index in multiple sclerosis. Cerebrospinal fluid IgM oligoclonal bands and clinical features to predict the evolution of the disease. Journal of Neurology. 2008;**255**:1023-1031

[59] Axelsson M, Malmeström C, Nilsson S, et al. Glial fibrillary acidic protein: A potential biomarker for progression in multiple sclerosis. Journal of Neurology. 2011;**258**:882-888

[60] Williams TE, Holdsworth KP, Nicholas JM, et al. Assessing Neurofilaments as biomarkers of neuroprotection in progressive multiple sclerosis: From the MS-STAT randomized controlled trial. NeurologyNeuroimmunology Neuroinflammation. 2022;**9**(2)

[61] Polman CH, Bertolotto A, Deisenhammer F, et al. Recommendations for clinical use of data on neutralising antibodies to interferon-beta therapy in multiple sclerosis. Lancet Neurology. 2010;**9**:740-750

[62] Gunnarsson M, Malmeström C, Axelsson M, et al. Axonal damage in relapsing multiple sclerosis is markedly reduced by natalizumab. Annals of Neurology. 2011;**69**:83-89

[63] Akgün K, Kretschmann N, Haase R, et al. Profiling individual clinical responses by high-frequency

serum neurofilament assessment in MS. Neurology: Neuroimmunology & Neuroinflammation. 2019;**6**:e555

[64] Villar LM, García-Sánchez MI, Costa-Frossard L, et al. Immunological markers of optimal response to natalizumab in multiple sclerosis. Archives of Neurology. 2012;**69**:191-197

[65] Galboiz Y, Shapiro S, Lahat N, et al. Matrix metalloproteinases and their tissue inhibitors as markers of disease subtype and response to interferon-beta therapy in relapsing and secondary-progressive multiple sclerosis patients. Annals of Neurology. 2001;**50**:443-451

[66] Bernal F, Elias B, Hartung HP, et al. Regulation of matrix metalloproteinases and their inhibitors by interferon-beta: A longitudinal study in multiple sclerosis patients. Multiple Sclerosis. 2009;**15**:721-727

[67] Comabella M, Río J, Espejo C, et al. Changes in matrix metalloproteinases and their inhibitors during interferon-beta treatment in multiple sclerosis. Clinical Immunology. 2009;**130**:145-150

[68] Balasa R, Bianca C, Septimiu V, et al. The matrix metalloproteinases panel in multiple sclerosis patients treated with Natalizumab: A possible answer to Natalizumab non-responders. CNS & Neurological Disorders Drug Targets. 2018;**17**:464-472

[69] Castellazzi M, Bellini T, Trentini A, et al. Serum gelatinases levels in multiple sclerosis patients during 21 months of Natalizumab therapy. Disease Markers. 2016;**2016**:8434209

[70] Fissolo N, Pignolet B, Matute-Blanch C, et al. Biomarkers and response to Natalizumab for multiple sclerosis treatment (BIONAT), best EScalation treatment in multiple sclerosis (BEST-MS), and the Société francophone de la Sclérose En plaques (SFSEP) network. Matrix metalloproteinase 9 is decreased in natalizumab-treated multiple sclerosis patients at risk for progressive multifocal leukoencephalopathy. Annals of Neurology. 2017;**82**:186-195

[71] Ibitoye R, Kemp K, Rice C, et al. Oxidative stress-related biomarkers in multiple sclerosis: A review. Biomarkers in Medicine. 2016;**10**:889-902

[72] Yuceyar N, Taşkiran D, Sağduyu A. Serum and cerebrospinal fluid nitrite and nitrate levels in relapsing-remitting and secondary progressive multiple sclerosis patients. Clinical Neurology and Neurosurgery. 2001;**103**:206-211

[73] Sellebjerg F, Giovannoni G, Hand A, et al. Cerebrospinal fluid levels of nitric oxide metabolites predict response to methylprednisolone treatment in multiple sclerosis and optic neuritis. Journal of Neuroimmunology. 2002;**125**:198-203

[74] Yamashita T, Ando Y, Obayashi K, et al. Changes in nitrite and nitrate (NO2-/NO3-) levels in cerebrospinal fluid of patients with multiple sclerosis. Journal of the Neurological Sciences. 1997;**153**:32-34

[75] Acar G, Idiman F, Idiman E, et al. Nitric oxide as an activity marker in multiple sclerosis. Journal of Neurology. 2003;**250**:588-592

[76] Rejdak K, Eikelenboom MJ, Petzold A, et al. CSF nitric oxide metabolites are associated with activity and progression of multiple sclerosis. Neurology. 2004;**63**:1439-1445

[77] Del Prete A, Scutera S, Sozzani S, et al. Role of osteopontin in dendritic cell shaping of immune responses. Cytokine & Growth Factor Reviews. 2019;**50**:19-28

[78] Murugaiyan G, Mittal A, Weiner HL. Increased osteopontin expression in dendritic cells amplifies IL-17 production by CD4+ T cells in experimental autoimmune encephalomyelitis and in multiple sclerosis. Journal of Immunology. 2008;**181**:7480-7488

[79] Braitch M, Constantinescu CS. The role of osteopontin in experimental autoimmune encephalomyelitis (EAE) and multiple sclerosis (MS). Inflammation & Allergy Drug Targets. 2010;**9**:249-256

[80] Sato W, Tomita A, Ichikawa D, et al. CCR2(+)CCR5(+) T cells produce matrix metalloproteinase-9 and osteopontin in the pathogenesis of multiple sclerosis. Journal of Immunology. 2012;**189**:5057-5065

[81] Chabas D, Baranzini SE, Mitchell D, et al. The influence of the proinflammatory cytokine, osteopontin, on autoimmune demyelinating disease. Science. 2001;**294**:1731-1735

[82] Londoño AC, Mora CA. Role of CXCL13 in the formation of the meningeal tertiary lymphoid organ in multiple sclerosis. F1000Research. 2018;**7**:514

[83] Krumbholz M, Theil D, Cepok S, et al. Chemokines in multiple sclerosis: CXCL12 and CXCL13 up-regulation is differentially linked to CNS immune cell recruitment. Brain. 2006;**129**:200-211

[84] Khademi M, Kockum I, Andersson ML, et al. Cerebrospinal fluid CXCL13 in multiple sclerosis: A suggestive prognostic marker for the disease course. Multiple Sclerosis. 2011;**17**:335-343

[85] Wang Y, Wu H, Wu X, et al. Interleukin 17A promotes gastric cancer invasiveness via NF-κB mediated matrix metalloproteinases 2 and 9 expression. PLoS One. 2014;**9**:e96678

[86] Trentini A, Castellazzi M, Cervellati C, et al. Interplay between matrix Metalloproteinase-9, matrix Metalloproteinase-2, and interleukins in multiple sclerosis patients. Disease Markers. 2016;**2016**:3672353

[87] Noppe M, Crols R, Andries D, et al. Determination in human cerebrospinal fluid of glial fibrillary acidic protein, S-100 and myelin basic protein as indices of nonspecific or specific central nervous tissue pathology. Clinica Chimica Acta. 1986;**155**:143-150

[88] Lamers KJ, de Reus HP, Jongen PJ. Myelin basic protein in CSF as indicator of disease activity in multiple sclerosis. Multiple Sclerosis. 1998;**4**:124-126

[89] Whitaker JN. Myelin encephalitogenic protein fragments in cerebrospinal fluid of persons with multiple sclerosis. Neurology. 1977;**27**:911-920

[90] Barkhof F, Frequin ST, Hommes OR, et al. A correlative triad of gadolinium-DTPA MRI, EDSS, and CSF-MBP in relapsing multiple sclerosis patients treated with high-dose intravenous methylprednisolone. Neurology. 1992;**42**:63-67

[91] Massaro AR. The role of NCAM in remyelination. Neurological Sciences. 2002;**22**:429-435

[92] Malmeström C, Haghighi S, Rosengren L, et al. Neurofilament light protein and glial fibrillary acidic protein as biological markers in MS. Neurology. 2003;**23**:1720-1725

[93] Matsushita T, Tateishi T, Isobe N, et al. Characteristic cerebrospinal fluid cytokine/chemokine profiles in neuromyelitis optica, relapsing remitting or primary progressive multiple sclerosis. PLoS One. 2013;**18**:e61835

[94] Virgilio E, Vecchio D, Crespi I, et al. Cerebrospinal fluid biomarkers and cognitive functions at multiple sclerosis diagnosis. Journal of Neurology. 2022:1-9

[95] Kuhle J, Nourbakhsh B, Grant D, et al. Serum neurofilament is associated with progression of brain atrophy and disability in early MS. Neurology. 2017;**88**:826-831

[96] Ferraro D, Trovati A, Bedin R, et al. Cerebrospinal fluid kappa and lambda free light chains in oligoclonal band negative patients with suspected multiple sclerosis. European Journal of Neurology. 2020;**27**:461-467

[97] Hayes DF. Biomarker validation and testing. Molecular Oncology. 2014;**9**:960-966

[98] Vermersch P, Berger T, Gold R, et al. The clinical perspective: How to personalise treatment in MS and how may biomarkers including imaging contribute to this? Multiple Sclerosis Journal. 2016;**22**:18-33

Chapter 3

Exploring the Effect of Genetic, Environmental and Lifestyle Factors on Multiple Sclerosis Susceptibility

Omar Deeb, Sawsan Salameh and Afnan Atallah

Abstract

Multiple sclerosis (MS) is a central nervous system inflammatory illness that begins with immune system dysregulation and impairs information flow inside the brain as well as between the brain and the rest of the body. The cause of MS is yet unknown. The interplay of genetic predispositions with environmental/lifestyle factors, such as smoking, obesity, viral exposure, and insufficient sun exposure, has led to numerous theories. This is reinforced by a major discovery of gene–environment (GxE) interaction, which could provide information on the disease's molecular pathways to aid in the identification of new therapy and preventative strategies, as well as steer disease exploration to new lifestyle suggestions. While some persons with the major susceptibility to MS have a human leukocyte antigen (HLA) Class II gene, according to genetic studies. We will cover recent studies relating to several genetic, environmental, and lifestyle factors, as well as their impact on MS, in this chapter.

Keywords: multiple sclerosis (MS), genetic factors, environment factors, lifestyle factors, human leukocyte antigen (HLA)

1. Introduction

Multiple sclerosis (MS) is a central nervous system (CNS) immune-mediated disease characterized by demyelination and gliosis as a result of immune cell infiltration across the blood–brain barrier. The disease's neurologic signs and symptoms are highly variable and dependent on the location of lesions in the CNS [1]. MS is the leading cause of non-traumatic disability in children. This disorder is a multifactorial, immune-mediated disease influenced by both genetic and environmental factors [2]. The prevalence of MS is expected to rise significantly in 2020, with an estimated 2.8 million people living with the disease worldwide in 2020, which is 30% more than in 2013, and it is more common in women than in men [3].

The exact cause of MS is unknown, but it is widely assumed that the disease is caused by complex gene–environment interactions [4, 5]. Genetic factors are important for characterizing pathogenetic mechanisms, and for elucidating the complex picture of disease initiation in the context of lifestyle and environmental factors Human leukocyte antigen (HLA) class I and II genes, which are the most strongly associated loci to MS. HLA class I and II genes encode for molecules that present antigens to CD4+ and CD8+ T lymphocytes [5]. In addition to genetic variants, lifestyle and environmental factors can be the important contributors to disease risk. Exposure to tobacco smoke and organic solvents, certain infections such as Epstein–Barr virus (EBV) infection, adolescent obesity, low levels of vitamin D and low exposure to sunlight, climate, and working night shifts are all risk factors (**Figure 1**), (**Table 1**). Use of oral tobacco, high coffee consumption, alcohol consumption, and serological evidence of cytomegalovirus (CMV) infection are all factors that may be associated with a lower risk (**Table 1**) [5–8].

MS risk and severity are influenced by a combination of genetic, environmental, and lifestyle/behavioral variables. This chapter explores the evidence regarding the impact of environmental and lifestyle factors such as sunshine and/or vitamin D,

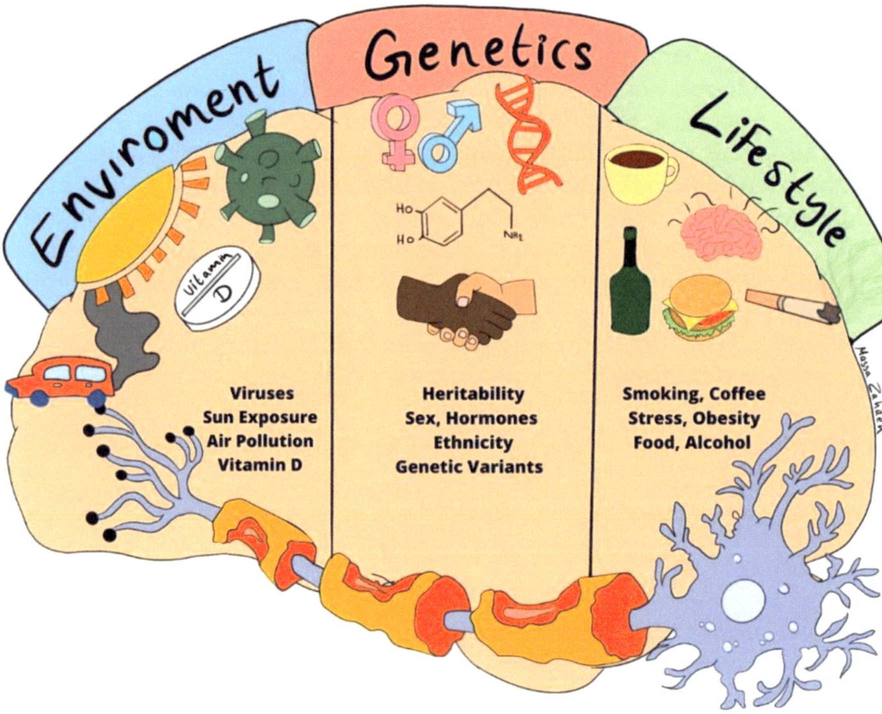

Figure 1.
The pathogenesis of multiple sclerosis is influenced by both genetic and environmental factors. Gender, disease-modifier genes, disease susceptibility genes, and single nucleotide polymorphisms are among the genetic factors that play a significant role in MS prevalence and pathogenesis. Environmental factors, on the other hand, such as smoking, vitamin D deficiency, exposure to pollutants, alcohol, diet style, Epstein Barr infection, dysbiosis of the gut microbiota, lack of exercise, and stress, are strongly linked to MS susceptibility and progression.

Factor	OR	HLA gene interaction	Combined OR	Immune system implied
Smoking	~1.5	Yes	14	yes
Oral tobacco	~0.5	ND	NA	yes
EBV infection (seropositivity)	~3.6	Yes	~16	yes
CMV infection (seropositivity)	~0.7	No	NA	yes
Work shift	~1.7	No	NA	yes
Adolescent obesity (BMI > 27)	~2	Yes	~15	Yes
Vitamin D level < 50 nM	~1.4	No	NA	Yes
Low sun exposure	~2	No	NA	Yes
Alcohol	~0.7–0.8	No	NA	Yes
Coffee	~0.7	No	NA	Yes

OR, Odd ratio; HLA, Human Leukocyte Antigen; EBV, Epstein–Barr virus; CMV, cytomegalovirus; BMI, body mass index; ND, not determined, NA, not applicable.

Table 1.
Summary of established and tentative lifestyle/environmental factors and their potential interactions with human leukocyte antigen (HLA) risk genes for multiple sclerosis (MS).

EBV infection, smoking and alcohol consumption, and other factors at various life stages, and addresses the issues in-depth and the impact of genetic variability on some.

2. Evidence for genetic factors

2.1 HLA-associated genetic variants

Human leukocyte antigen (HLA) class I and II genes are particularly important disease risk modifiers: class II gene variants encode products that present antigens to CD4+ T lymphocytes, while class I products present antigens to CD8+ lymphocytes. The class II variant HLADRB1*15: 01 is a risk allele of MS (odds ratio (OR) ~3) and is carried by 25–30% of the population in northern Europe and the United States. The second most powerful MS gene, class I variant HLAA*02, is associated with a lower risk of MS (OR ~0.6). While the absence of HLAA*02 combined with the presence of DRB1*15: 01 has a combined OR of ~5 [5, 9–12].

Several cohort studies suggest that the HLA genotype can influence environmental influences on MS risk. The harmful effects of childhood obesity [13], smoking [14–16], infectious mononucleosis, and solvent exposure [16] on MS risk are amplified in those who carry the HLA DRB1*15 allele and lack the protective HLA A*02 genotype. A recent study found a strong link between higher childhood body mass index (BMI) at age 10, smoking before the age of 20, and earlier menarche and MS. In a combined model that included the HLA DRB1*15:01 and HLA A*02:01 genotypes, the effects of these three risk factors remained similar [6]. Environmental risk factors have been shown to play an important role in the development of MS disease in genetically susceptible populations (class II HLA-DRB1*15:01 carriers) [17].

3. Environmental factors

3.1 Past viral infections

3.1.1 Epstein-Barr virus (EBV)

The mechanisms by which previous viral infections and viral reactivation may contribute to MS onset are still unknown. Epstein-Barr virus (EBV) is one of these viruses that has been linked to an increased risk of MS, as it has been discovered that people who have had clinically overt infectious mononucleosis (IM) have a more than twofold risk of developing MS [18, 19]. This organization has recently received funding. According to a longitudinal study, the risk of MS increased 32-fold after infection with EBV but not after infection with other viruses [20]. Supporting the link between EBV and MS, EBV-induced infectious mononucleosis, positivity for EBV nuclear antigen (EBNA)-1 IgG, or higher EBNA-1 titers have all been linked to an increased risk of MS (OR ~3.6) [21, 22]. Furthermore, there appears to be a critical time window for EBV infection, with infection occurring during adolescence or later implying an increased risk of developing MS, whereas this is not the case in childhood [23].

The genetic risk for elevated antiEBNA1 titers has been found to be positively correlated with the development of MS [24], which could be interpreted as additional evidence for EBV's causality in MS. It has been reported that EBNA positivity interacts with both HLA-A*02 and HLA-DRB1*15 [25, 26]. Another study of MS cases and healthy non-MS controls who were seropositive for EBV found that HLA-A*A02-positive individuals had the lowest EBV viral load and HLA-DRB1*15-positive individuals had the highest. These findings support EBV's causal role in MS, which is modulated by the HLA Class 1 genotype via changes in antigen presentation to T cells [27]. It has also been reported that an additive interaction of EBV status with HLA DRB1*15:01 modifies MS risk [28, 29]. People who tested positive for HLA-DRB1 *15, negative for HLA-A* 02, and had high EBNA-1 titers, had a 16-fold increased risk of MS compared to those who did not carry any of these factors, with a combined OR of ~16 [26].

The genetic risk for elevated antiEBNA1 titers is positively correlated with the development of MS, which could be further evidence for EBV causality in MS [24]. Infectious mononucleosis and increased EBNA1 antibody titers interact with HLA MS risk genetic variants [26]; and infectious mononucleosis interacts with HLA DRB1*15:01 [30] to increase the risk of MS in a pattern similar to smoking. Because HLA risk alleles encode molecules that regulate T cell adaptive immunity, the interaction with EBV infection measures may point to common pathogenetic pathways in MS [5].

3.1.2 Cytomegalovirus (CMV)

Cytomegalovirus (CMV) is a herpes virus that is related to EBV. CMV infection is mostly asymptomatic. Multiple studies have found a negative correlation between CMV seropositivity and MS diagnosis (protective association) in both pediatric and adult populations, with an OR of ~0.7 [31–35]. While a few studies have failed to find a link between CMV seropositivity and MS risk [36–38],

CMV infection may have a potentially protective effect due to its ability to induce not only pro-inflammatory antiviral responses, but also several anti-inflammatory responses, such as decreased mononuclear cell proliferation, increased anti-inflammatory cytokine secretion, and decreased cell surface HLA class I and II expression [31]. CMV infection alters the phenotype and function of B cells in MS, modulating the influence of IFN and reducing the proinflammatory B cell profile, according to new research. These findings may help to explain the potential impact of this viral infection on MS [39].

3.1.3 Herpes simplex virus (HSV)

Controversial findings regarding the relationship between HSV infection and MS risk [40–42]. According to a new study, HSV infection is modestly associated with MS risk, particularly in Whites, raising the possibility that the disparity between previous reports is due to the racial make-up of study populations [29]. This study also confirmed the link between HLADRB1 status, HSV infection, and the risk of MS. HSV infection was linked to an increased risk of MS only in HLA-DRB1*15:01 negative subjects [29, 32].

3.2 Sun exposure/Vitamin

There are large number of studies on sun exposure/vitamin D, provoked by epidemiologic observations of a latitude-dependent difference in MS incidence and prevalence, despite being confounded by the distribution of the HLA DRB1*15:01 risk predisposing genotype in gradients [43, 44].

Because we rely on ultraviolet radiation (UVR) to convert vitamin D to an active metabolite, distinguishing the effect of UVR from that of vitamin D is difficult. Both of these exposures have been linked to a lower risk of MS, according to a recent and extensive review [45]. A higher level of UVR exposure is associated with a lower risk of MS [43, 46, 47]. Even after accounting for vitamin D levels, there was still a link between UVR exposure habits and the risk of MS [47], though this finding should be interpreted with caution because vitamin D levels were not measured prior to the preclinical phase. The physiological reason for UVR's putative protective impact is still being researched. UVR exposure protects against MS even if vitamin D isn't present. When tested in the animal model EAE [48], UVR exposure lowers peripheral inflammation in mice [49], with a T regulatory (Treg) cell activation and dampening effects on antigen-presenting dendritic cells [50, 51]. In these instances, cis-uronic acid production could be involved [52].

Increased vitamin D levels have been linked to a lower incidence of MS, particularly before the age of 20 [53], which is consistent with later results on supplementation and sun exposure [54, 55]. Furthermore, in the situation of minimal sunlight exposure, a diet rich in vitamin D containing fatty fish reduces MS risk [56]. In one study of vitamin D levels during pregnancy in humans using birth samples, no difference between MS cases and controls was found; despite large confidence intervals [57], which is consistent with studies on experimental autoimmune encephalomyelitis (EAE) in which only adolescent rats (not pregnancy or adult rats) showed an effect of vitamin D [58]. This discovery is not without controversy, as mothers with low vitamin D levels during the first trimester had a two-fold greater risk of MS in their offspring [59]. Variations in sampling timing, storing issues, or possible "inherited" behavior differences regarding sun exposure are all possible explanations for the disparate results. In Australia, epidemiologic studies of sun exposure found a link between low sun exposure in mothers during the first trimester and the risk of MS in their children [60]. Regardless, vitamin D and/or sun exposure appear to be significant during a temporal window of adolescence when vitamin supplementation may reduce MS risk to some extent. Vitamin D's importance is also confirmed by genetic data, which shows that mutations around the CYP27B1 gene, which is involved in vitamin D metabolism, are linked to MS [61, 62]. In two case-control investigations, recent genomic data on a series of genes that regulate Vitamin D levels revealed significant effects. Because the distribution of these gene variants is random, it resembles a blinded clinical trial or Mendelian randomization in certain ways [63, 64]. In vitro investigations using the biggest MS risk gene, HLA DRB1*15:01, identified vitamin D as the first example of a gene–environment interaction [65], although this finding has not been replicated in humans [47].

It is still unclear whether vitamin D or sun exposure has a strong therapeutic effect once MS has been diagnosed. Despite the fact that vitamin D has been introduced to conventional therapy in multiple research, its value has yet to be determined. Importantly, high vitamin D levels are linked to reduced axonal injury as evaluated by cerebrospinal fluid (CSF), neurofilament light [66], and greater vitamin D levels were linked to lower MRI activity and delayed disease development during an interferon study [67, 68].

Vitamin D supplementation is thought to be non-toxic even at very high doses, so it seems reasonable to conduct large clinical trials in people at risk for MS, such as close relatives, or even to recommend supplementation at relatively high doses for all adolescents; vitamin D appears to play a role in a variety of diseases, not just MS. Because of the risk of skin cancer, it is more difficult to make sun exposure recommendations. Moderate exposure, on the other hand, is a good idea. Variations in the timing of sample, storage challenges, or possible "inherited" behavior variances towards sun exposure are all plausible causes for the lack of consensus on whether vitamin D supplementation is beneficial in individuals. Notably, epidemiologic studies of sun exposure in Australia found evidence of a link between low sun exposure in mothers and the development of MS. Many MS patients, on the other hand, are aware of the link between vitamin D and MS risk and take it, especially during the winter.

3.3 Air pollution

The link between air pollutant exposure and MS risk is unclear. Particulate matter (PM) exposure causes an inflammatory response in the lung, resulting in the release of inflammatory cytokines and elevated systemic levels. Long-term exposure to air pollution has been linked to neuroinflammation and blood–brain barrier damage. Studies examining exposure to particles with an aerodynamic diameter of less than10 μm (PM10) produced conflicting results [69–71]. Seasonal exposure to nitrogen dioxide during the cold season or ozone during the hot season has been linked to an increased risk of MS relapse, whereas exposure to benzene and carbon monoxide was not [72].

4. Lifestyle factors

4.1 Smoking and oral tobacco

Cigarette smoking is a well-established risk factor for MS (OR of 1.5) [73, 74]; this finding result was later confirmed in a larger case-control study [75, 76], with a clear dose-response relationship [76, 77]; cumulative smoking is associated with an increase in risk [15, 75, 78, 79]. Elevated levels of cotinine in the serum or plasma (≥ 10 ng/ml) from patients before they developed MS were associated with a significantly increased risk of MS (OR of 1.5). The effect on the risk for MS by cotinine levels was significant in individuals younger than 26 years old with OR of 2.2 [80]. However, the age at which a person first began smoking had no effect on the association between smoking and MS risk [76]. Passive smoking exposure, including water pipe smoking, but not oral tobacco use in the form of moist snuff, has also been linked to an increased risk of MS [14, 81]. Also, children raised in environments associated with smoker parents had more than double the risk of a first MS episode when compared with unexposed children, this increase in risk was significantly associated with the longer duration of exposure [82]. In addition, children exposed to second-hand smoke and with HLA-DBR1*15 alleles have a higher risk of MS [83], implying that even minor lung irritation is significant [84]. If the association is due to nonspecific irritation, one might consider a factor such as air pollution as a trigger of CNS neuroinflammation, as long-term exposure to air pollutants has been confirmed as an environmental risk factor in MS [69]. On the other hand, smoking increases risk of developing neutralizing antibodies against some MS treatments, such as natalizumab and interferon β [85, 86].

Oral tobacco reduces the risk of developing MS in a dose-dependent manner [75, 87]. Nicotine may have such a protective effect due to its agonistic effect on the alpha 7 subunit of acetylcholine, expressed on the surface of CD4(+) T cells [88]. This finding lends credence to the idea that, despite nicotine's apparent protective effects, it is lung inflammation that drives the increase in risk.

Smoking has a remarkable interaction with HLA risk genes associated with MS. In the Scandinavian population, carriers of the HLA DRB1*15:01 confer an OR of 3, and lack of HLA-A*02 confers an OR of ~1.8, resulting in a combined OR of 5 among nonsmokers; however, among smokers, the combined OR is ~14, much higher than the sum of the main effects associated with each factor [15]. In studies of passive smoke exposure, such a gene–environment interaction has been replicated [14]. These findings indicate a strong link between HLA genotypes and disease development [89].

Smoking also interacts with a non-HLA gene variant, the N-Acetyltransferase 1 (NAT1) gene (gene encoding the N-acetyltransferase 1 enzyme, which is important in the metabolism of aromatic amines present in cigarette smoke), as smokers with NAT1 single nucleotide polymorphisms are at a higher risk of developing MS [90]. As a result, the impact of smoking is highly dependent on genetic context [5, 7].

4.2 Obesity and body mass index

Female adolescent obesity has been linked to MS in large cohorts [91]. It has been found that adolescent obesity was associated with an OR of ~2 in both males and females, despite the fact that adult body mass index (BMI) at diagnosis had no effect [13]. The link is highest with a BMI of > 27, but increased ORs can be seen at lower BMI levels as well. Obesity has been linked to a higher incidence of MS in children [91, 92]. It has been discovered that the critical period for adult MS appears to be during adolescence rather than at the age of ten [93]. A Norwegian/Italian study published results that were very comparable [94]. Furthermore, Mendelian randomization studies reveal that genetic determinants for high BMI are related to an increased risk of MS, despite several possible confounders and biases attributed to reverse causation, indicating that this lifestyle factor plays a causative role [64, 95].

In this scenario, there is also an interaction with MS HLA risk genes; specifically, DRB1*15:01 positive and HLA A*02 negative persons with a high BMI have an OR of ~14 [13], indicating that biological pathways are shared and that obesity is a causal factor. Even however, the underlying mechanistic routes are still unknown. At the very least, we evaluate three non-exclusive and somewhat overlapping pathways: (1) Obesity is associated with "low-grade" inflammation, in which fat tissue produces higher quantities of proinflammatory mediators [96, 97]. Promotion of T helper (Th) 1-biased immune responses and decreased function of Treg cells have been described [98]; (2) In the presence of obesity, increased levels of leptin, a mediator connected to proinflammation, are observed [99]; (3) Obesity also leads to decreased bioavailability of vitamin D, in turn with options for a pro-inflammatory bias [100]. Any of the potential mechanisms may enhance the activation and functional proinflammatory bias of adaptive autoreactive immune cells, which may cause the neuroinflammatory bouts, a sequence of events that is supported by the HLA gene interaction; HLA genes encode the antigen-presenting molecules necessary for activation of T cells.

The observed interaction between EBV/IM and BMI, acting independently of the HLA DRB1*15:01 class II risk allele, where each of the two lifestyle/environmental factors results in ORs of 2, but approaches 14 when combined, strongly supports the relevance of obesity with regard to a putative immune attack on the CNS [101]. The causes for the interaction are still unknown. Obesity is linked to a less effective immune response to infections in general, so it's possible that obesity will result in a less effective immune response to EBV [102, 103]. It's also possible that a combined proinflammatory environment during obesity, as well as the as-yet-undefined effects of EBV linked to MS, are exacerbating the risk of neuroinflammation. Our argument is based on the fact that there is an interaction between EBV and obesity, two MS risk factors, in the development of MS, supporting the idea that both of them play a causal role in triggering onset.

Obesity data and MS may have a direct link with prevention in this scenario, especially for those who are at high risk for MS, such as children or other relatives of people with MS. It's also relevant to the global obesity pandemic, and it could be one of the factors contributing to the rise in MS cases among women around the world.

4.3 Alcohol consumption

A number of research have been carried out to look into the role of alcohol in MS. There was evidence indicating a dose-dependent inverse connection between MS and alcohol in two large case-control studies, with ORs in the range of 0.7–0.8 [104]. Low and moderate alcohol use has been demonstrated to lower innate inflammatory responses in humans [105–107], which is consistent with recent data that show alcohol consumption is negatively related to MS risk. In terms of MS risk, it has been discovered that the existence of DRB1*15:01 and non-drinking, as well as smoking and non-drinking, have interactions [108].

Although still significant, the relationship between non-drinking and smoking was less prominent among previous smokers than among current smokers. This finding may not come as a surprise, given the long-term negative impact of smoking on MS risk after quitting [76]. Interleukin-21 is a major immune modulator that may enhance autoimmune responses through various mechanisms such as the development and activation of helper T-17 and follicular helper T cells, as well as the suppression of regulatory T cells [109], which has been shown to be reduced by alcohol and its metabolite acetate. Interleukin-21 has been linked to the onset of a number of autoimmune illnesses and has also been linked to the severity and progression of MS [110, 111].

Due to preexisting detrimental effects on CNS by the MS process, individuals may experience decreased alcohol tolerance and so restrict their alcohol consumption before the beginning of MS. Alcohol intake, on the other hand, has been linked to an increased risk of various autoimmune illnesses that do not directly damage the CNS [112–114]. Furthermore, alcohol use throughout adolescence was linked to a decreased incidence of MS [115] in a recent Danish case–control study.

To summarize, non-drinkers have a higher risk of developing MS than drinkers, and non-drinking combines with DRB1*15:01 and smoking to raise disease risk. Alcohol use has been shown to have negative effects on other disease conditions, and a greater understanding of the mechanisms behind our findings may aid in the development of new approaches to guard against MS without using alcohol.

4.4 Coffee consumption

Only a few studies have looked at the effects of coffee consumption on the risk and severity of MS, in contrast to the intense interest in the effects of smoking. Two independent population-based case-control studies recently looked into the link between coffee consumption and MS risk. The risk of MS was significantly lowered in individuals who reported drinking more than 900 mL of coffee per day (OR 0.70) [116]. In a case–control research with 93 cases and 186 controls, of which 92 were hospital controls and 94 were population controls, persons who took coffee before the age of 15 years had a higher risk of MS; however, there was no link between MS risk and coffee consumption beyond that age [117]. Increased coffee consumption was linked to an increased incidence of MS in a hospital-based case–control research with 210 incident cases and 210 individually matched controls. The inverse relationship between coffee drinking and the beginning of chronic diseases such as cardiovascular disease, diabetes, Parkinson's disease, and various malignancies has led the US Dietary Guidelines Advisory Committee to suggest moderate coffee consumption as part of a healthy diet [118]. Coffee drinking could play a role in MS through a number of different processes. Caffeine therapy protects against experimental autoimmune encephalomyelitis by increasing the number of adenosine 1A receptors [119, 120]. In addition, caffeine administration of human monocytoid cells in vitro boosted the expression of adenosine 1A receptors while lowering pro-inflammatory cytokine output [121]. Although this study was cross-sectional, a causal relationship could not be verified, coffee drinking has also been linked to a slower progression of disability in relapsing onset MS [122]. More research is needed to determine whether the findings are due to caffeine or another molecule in coffee, to longitudinally assess the association between coffee consumption and MS disease activity, and to evaluate the mechanisms by which coffee may act, which could lead to new therapeutic targets.

4.5 Diet

The experimental findings regarding immune system modulation by salt concentration have been validated. In vitro studies suggest that lower intracellular sodium concentrations and sodium intake may have immune-protective effects [123–125]. While a large epidemiological study aimed at determining the relationship between dietary sodium intake and MS found that neither baseline energy-adjusted sodium levels nor cumulative longitudinal sodium intake was associated with an increased risk of developing MS [126, 127]. Other studies sought to determine the effect of salt consumption on the ongoing disease process, as it has been reported that individuals with MS who consumed a lot of salt had a lot more relapses and magnetic resonance imaging (MRI) evidenced disease activity than those who ate less salt [128]. On the contrary, studies that looked at patients' sodium urine excretion levels found no correlation with conversion to clinically definite MS, nor with clinical or MRI outcomes over a five-year period [127]. The same results have been shown in the pediatric MS population [129, 130].

The relationship between polyunsaturated fatty acids (PUFAs) and MS has been investigated. Several studies [56, 131, 132] found that a higher intake of total PUFA at baseline was associated with a lower risk of MS. Clinical trials, on the other hand, have found no effect of a low-fat diet on relapse rate or MRI activity [133]. Furthermore, omega-3 supplementation had no effect on disease activity [134]. A higher saturated fat intake was associated with higher relapse risk in children with MS, whereas vegetable intake may be an independent protective factor [135].

In experimental MS models, the effects of various dietary changes have been studied (i.e., experimental autoimmune encephalomyelitis [EAE]). When compared to mice fed a normal diet, mice fed a high-fat diet showed increased gene expression of renin–angiotensin aldosterone system (RAAS) brain components, which coincided with increased vascular endothelial permeability, recruitment of inflammatory cells, upregulation of adhesion molecules, more severe exacerbations, and higher mean disease scores. The use of captopril which acts as an angiotensin-converting enzyme (ACE) inhibitor improves the outcomes of EAE disease [136]. A high-fat diet has also been linked to increased brain inflammation, decreased protective neurotrophic factors, and decreased neural plasticity, all of which impair learning and memory functions [137]. The EAE RAAS studies have proposed cardiovascular health as a potential link between dietary changes and MS outcomes by indicating a high-fat diet as a factor in MS [138].

4.6 Work shift

The relationship between shift work (night work) and MS has been studied. Shift work during adolescence (before the age of 20 years) has been shown to increase the risk of MS (OR ~1.7). Other studies [139–141] have confirmed these findings. These findings highlight the importance of melatonin in the disease. Shift work consequences, such as circadian disruption and sleep restriction, have been linked to disturbed melatonin secretion and increased proinflammatory responses, and may thus be part of the mechanism underlying the association [139, 142]. Avoiding night shift work, especially in people at high risk of MS, is another modifiable lifestyle factor that may help prevent the disease [5].

4.7 Gut microbiota

The composition and abundance of microbes in the intestinal microbiota are risk factors for the development of MS. MS in humans can be caused by changes in certain microbial populations in the gastrointestinal tract. Furthermore, the gut microbiota promotes an anti-inflammatory and protective environment capable of inhibiting the growth of pathogenic microorganisms that cause a variety of diseases [143, 144]. Furthermore, many factors, such as diet, obesity, antibiotic use, cigarette smoking, and stress, influence the gut microbiota and may influence the risk and/or course of MS [144]. The gut microbiota appears to be crucial in the pathogenesis of MS. It appears to be involved in immune system modulation, changes the integrity and function of biological barriers (blood–brain barrier), has a direct effect on several types of central nervous system-resident cells, and causes autoimmune demyelination [144, 145].

5. Conclusion

The influence of lifestyle/environmental factors on MS is becoming clearer. Combining genetics and environmental factors has aided the understanding of MS; factors interacting with MS risk genes, primarily HLA risk genes, can be argued to share etiologic pathways underlying the disease, as well as their effect on the immune system. This is true for adolescent obesity, tobacco use, and EBV infection. The understanding method is still in its early stages, but the vast majority of recognized factors may be related to immune system impacts, comparable to hereditary predisposing factors, implying that the peripheral immune system plays a critical role in MS. Factors that cause disease are increasingly being incorporated into practical health treatment and even prevention, particularly for people at high risk of MS, especially if the disease runs in the family.

Acknowledgements

Acknowledgment to our student Massa Zahdeh (massa.zahdeh@students.alquds.edu) in the faculty of pharmacy/Al-Quds University for drawing the figure.

Conflict of interest

The authors declare no conflict of interest.

Author details

Omar Deeb[1]*, Sawsan Salameh[1] and Afnan Atallah[2]

1 Faculty of Pharmacy, Al-Quds University, Jerusalem, Palestine

2 Faculty of Medicine, Al-Quds University, Jerusalem, Palestine

*Address all correspondence to: deeb.omar@gmail.com

References

[1] Agius MA, Klodowska-Duda G, Maciejowski M, et al. Safety and tolerability of inebilizumab (MEDI-551), an anti-CD19 monoclonal antibody, in patients with relapsing forms of multiple sclerosis: Results from a phase 1 randomised, placebo-controlled, escalating intravenous and subcutaneous dose study. Multiple Sclerosis. 2019;**25**:235-245

[2] Filippi M, Bar-Or A, Piehl F, et al. Multiple sclerosis. Nature Reviews Disease Primers. 2018;**4**:43

[3] Walton C, King R, Rechtman L, et al. Rising prevalence of multiple sclerosis worldwide: Insights from the Atlas of MS, third edition. Multiple Sclerosis. 2020;**26**:1816-1821

[4] Hecker M, Bühring J, Fitzner B, et al. Genetic, environmental and lifestyle determinants of accelerated telomere attrition as contributors to risk and severity of multiple sclerosis. Biomolecules. 2021;**11**:1510

[5] Olsson T, Barcellos LF, Alfredsson L. Interactions between genetic, lifestyle and environmental risk factors for multiple sclerosis. Nature Reviews. Neurology. 2017;**13**:25-36

[6] Jacobs BM, Noyce AJ, Bestwick J, Belete D, Giovannoni G, Dobson R. Gene-environment interactions in multiple sclerosis: A UK biobank study. Neurology: Neuroimmunology and NeuroInflammation. 28 May 2021;**8**(4):e1007. DOI: 10.1212/NXI.0000000000001007. PMID: 34049995; PMCID: PMC8192056

[7] Alfredsson L, Olsson T. Lifestyle and environmental factors in multiple sclerosis. Cold Spring Harbor Perspectives in Medicine. 2019;**9**:a028944

[8] Tobin O. Multiple Sclerosis - Symptoms and Causes [Internet]. Mayo Clinic. Available from: https://www.mayoclinic.org/diseases-conditions/multiple-sclerosis/symptoms-causes/syc-20350269 [cited 2022 Feb 10]

[9] Sawcer S, Hellenthal G, Pirinen M, et al. Genetic risk and a primary role for cell-mediated immune mechanisms in multiple sclerosis. Nature. 2011;**476**:214-219

[10] Brynedal B, Duvefelt K, Jonasdottir G, et al. HLA-A confers an HLA-DRB1 independent influence on the risk of multiple sclerosis. PLoS One. 2007;**2**:e664

[11] Moutsianas L, Jostins L, Beecham AH, et al. Class II HLA interactions modulate genetic risk for multiple sclerosis. Nature Genetics. 2015;**47**:1107-1113

[12] Waubant E, Lucas R, Mowry E, et al. Environmental and genetic risk factors for MS: An integrated review. Annals of Clinical Translational Neurology. 2019;**6**:1905-1922

[13] Hedström AK, Lima Bomfim I, Barcellos L, et al. Interaction between adolescent obesity and HLA risk genes in the etiology of multiple sclerosis. Neurology. 2014;**82**:865-872

[14] Hedström AK, Bomfim IL, Barcellos LF, et al. Interaction between passive smoking and two HLA genes with regard to multiple sclerosis risk. International Journal of Epidemiology. 2014;**43**:1791-1798

[15] Hedström AK, Sundqvist E, Bäärnhielm M, et al. Smoking and two human leukocyte antigen genes interact to increase the risk for multiple sclerosis. Brain. 2011;**134**:653-664

[16] Hedström AK, Hössjer O, Katsoulis M, et al. Organic solvents and MS susceptibility: Interaction with MS risk HLA genes. Neurology. 2018;**91**:e455-e462

[17] Goodin DS, Khankhanian P, Gourraud P-A, et al. The nature of genetic and environmental susceptibility to multiple sclerosis. PLoS One. 2021;**16**:e0246157

[18] Handel AE, Williamson AJ, Disanto G, et al. An updated meta-analysis of risk of multiple sclerosis following infectious mononucleosis. PLoS One. 2010;**5**:e12496

[19] Robinson WH, Steinman L. Epstein-Barr virus and multiple sclerosis. Science. 2022;**375**:264-265

[20] Bjornevik K, Cortese M, Healy BC, et al. Longitudinal analysis reveals high prevalence of Epstein-Barr virus associated with multiple sclerosis. Science. 2022;**375**:296-301

[21] Geginat J, Paroni M, Pagani M, et al. The enigmatic role of viruses in multiple sclerosis: Molecular mimicry or disturbed immune surveillance? Trends in Immunology. 2017;**38**:498-512

[22] Belbasis L, Bellou V, Evangelou E, et al. Environmental risk factors and multiple sclerosis: An umbrella review of systematic reviews and meta-analyses. Lancet Neurology. 2015;**14**:263-273

[23] Ascherio A, Munger KL. EBV and autoimmunity. Current Topics in Microbiology and Immunology. 2015;**390**:365-385

[24] Zhou Y, Zhu G, Charlesworth JC, et al. Genetic loci for Epstein-Barr virus nuclear antigen-1 are associated with risk of multiple sclerosis. Multiple Sclerosis. 2016;**22**:1655-1664

[25] Lucas RM, Ponsonby A-L, Dear K, et al. Current and past Epstein-Barr virus infection in risk of initial CNS demyelination. Neurology. 2011;**77**:371-379

[26] Sundqvist E, Sundström P, Lindén M, et al. Epstein-Barr virus and multiple sclerosis: Interaction with HLA. Genes and Immunity. 2012;**13**:14-20

[27] Agostini S, Mancuso R, Guerini FR, et al. HLA alleles modulate EBV viral load in multiple sclerosis. Journal of Translational Medicine. 2018;**16**:80

[28] Xiao D, Ye X, Zhang N, et al. A meta-analysis of interaction between Epstein-Barr virus and HLA-DRB1*1501 on risk of multiple sclerosis. Scientific Reports. 2015;**5**:18083

[29] Nourbakhsh B, Rutatangwa A, Waltz M, et al. Heterogeneity in association of remote herpesvirus infections and pediatric MS. Annals of Clinical Translational Neurology. 2018;**5**:1222-1228

[30] Nielsen TR, Rostgaard K, Askling J, et al. Effects of infectious mononucleosis and HLA-DRB1*15 in multiple sclerosis. Multiple Sclerosis. 2009;**15**:431-436

[31] Makhani N, Banwell B, Tellier R, et al. Viral exposures and MS outcome in a prospective cohort of children with acquired demyelination. Multiple Sclerosis. 2016;**22**:385-388

[32] Waubant E, Mowry EM, Krupp L, et al. Common viruses associated with lower pediatric multiple sclerosis risk. Neurology. 2011;**76**:1989-1995

[33] Sundqvist E, Bergström T, Daialhosein H, et al. Cytomegalovirus seropositivity is negatively associated with multiple sclerosis. Multiple Sclerosis. 2014;**20**:165-173

[34] Langer-Gould A, Wu J, Lucas R, et al. Epstein-Barr virus, cytomegalovirus, and multiple sclerosis susceptibility: A multiethnic study. Neurology. 2017;**89**:1330-1337

[35] Grut V, Biström M, Salzer J, et al. Cytomegalovirus seropositivity is associated with reduced risk of multiple sclerosis—A presymptomatic case–control study. European Journal of Neurology. 2021;**28**:3072-3079

[36] Ascherio A, Munger KL, Lennette ET, et al. Epstein-Barr virus antibodies and risk of multiple sclerosis: A Prospective Study. Journal of the American Medical Association. 2001;**286**:3083-3088

[37] DeLorenze GN, Munger KL, Lennette ET, et al. Epstein-Barr virus and multiple sclerosis: Evidence of association from a prospective study with long-term follow-up. Archives of Neurology. 2006;**63**:839-844

[38] Levin LI, Munger KL, Rubertone MV, et al. Temporal relationship between elevation of Epstein-Barr virus antibody titers and initial onset of neurological symptoms in multiple sclerosis. Journal of the American Medical Association. 2005;**293**:2496-2500

[39] Zabalza A, Vera A, Alari-Pahissa E, et al. Impact of cytomegalovirus infection on B cell differentiation and cytokine production in multiple sclerosis. Journal of Neuroinflammation. 2020;**17**:161

[40] Krone B, Pohl D, Rostasy K, et al. Common infectious agents in multiple sclerosis: A case—control study in children. Multiple Sclerosis. 2008;**14**:136-139

[41] MacGregor HS, Latiwonk QI. Complex role of gamma-herpesviruses in multiple sclerosis and infectious mononucleosis. Neurological Research. 1993;**15**:391-394

[42] Simmons A. Herpesvirus and multiple sclerosis. Herpes. 2001;**8**:60-63

[43] Simpson S, Blizzard L, Otahal P, et al. Latitude is significantly associated with the prevalence of multiple sclerosis: A meta-analysis. Journal of Neurology, Neurosurgery, and Psychiatry. 2011;**82**:1132-1141

[44] Koch-Henriksen N, Sørensen PS. The changing demographic pattern of multiple sclerosis epidemiology. Lancet Neurology. 2010;**9**:520-532

[45] Lucas RM, Byrne SN, Correale J, et al. Ultraviolet radiation, vitamin D and multiple sclerosis. Neurodegeneration Disease Management. 2015;**5**:413-424

[46] Kampman MT, Wilsgaard T, Mellgren SI. Outdoor activities and diet in childhood and adolescence relate to MS risk above the Arctic Circle. Journal of Neurology. 2007;**254**:471-477

[47] Bäärnhielm M, Hedström AK, Kockum I, et al. Sunlight is associated with decreased multiple sclerosis risk: No interaction with human leukocyte antigen-DRB1*15. European Journal of Neurology. 2012;**19**:955-962

[48] Becklund BR, Severson KS, Vang SV, et al. UV radiation suppresses experimental autoimmune encephalomyelitis independent of vitamin D production. Proceedings of the National Academy of Sciences of the United States of America. 2010;**107**:6418-6423

[49] Rana S, Rogers LJ, Halliday GM. Systemic low-dose UVB inhibits CD8 T cells and skin inflammation by alternative and novel mechanisms.

The American Journal of Pathology. 2011;**178**:2783-2791

[50] Navid F, Bruhs A, Schuller W, et al. The Aryl hydrocarbon receptor is involved in UVR-induced immunosuppression. The Journal of Investigative Dermatology. 2013;**133**:2763-2770

[51] Breuer J, Schwab N, Schneider-Hohendorf T, et al. Ultraviolet B light attenuates the systemic immune response in central nervous system autoimmunity. Annals of Neurology. 2014;**75**:739-758

[52] Correale J, Farez MF. Modulation of multiple sclerosis by sunlight exposure: Role of cis-urocanic acid. Journal of Neuroimmunology. 2013;**261**:134-140

[53] Munger KL, Levin LI, Hollis BW, et al. Serum 25-hydroxyvitamin D levels and risk of multiple sclerosis. Journal of the American Medical Association. 2006;**296**:2832-2838

[54] Bjørnevik K, Riise T, Casetta I, et al. Sun exposure and multiple sclerosis risk in Norway and Italy: The EnvIMS study. Multiple Sclerosis. 2014;**20**:1042-1049

[55] Cortese M, Riise T, Bjørnevik K, et al. Timing of use of cod liver oil, a vitamin D source, and multiple sclerosis risk: The EnvIMS study. Multiple Sclerosis. 2015;**21**:1856-1864

[56] Bäärnhielm M, Olsson T, Alfredsson L. Fatty fish intake is associated with decreased occurrence of multiple sclerosis. Multiple Sclerosis. 2014;**20**:726-732

[57] Ueda P, Rafatnia F, Bäärnhielm M, et al. Neonatal vitamin D status and risk of multiple sclerosis. Annals of Neurology. 2014;**76**:338-346

[58] Adzemovic MZ, Zeitelhofer M, Hochmeister S, et al. Efficacy of vitamin D in treating multiple sclerosis-like neuroinflammation depends on developmental stage. Experimental Neurology. 2013;**249**:39-48

[59] Munger KL, Åivo J, Hongell K, et al. Vitamin D status during pregnancy and risk of multiple sclerosis in Offspring of Women in the Finnish Maternity Cohort. JAMA Neurology. 2016;**73**:515-519

[60] Staples J, Ponsonby A-L, Lim L. Low maternal exposure to ultraviolet radiation in pregnancy, month of birth, and risk of multiple sclerosis in offspring: Longitudinal analysis. BMJ. 2010;**340**:c1640

[61] International Multiple Sclerosis Genetics Consortium (IMSGC), Beecham AH, Patsopoulos NA, et al. Analysis of immune-related loci identifies 48 new susceptibility variants for multiple sclerosis. Nature Genetics. 2013;**45**:1353-1360

[62] Sundqvist E, Bäärnhielm M, Alfredsson L, et al. Confirmation of association between multiple sclerosis and CYP27B1. European Journal of Human Genetics. 2010;**18**:1349-1352

[63] Mokry LE, Ross S, Ahmad OS, et al. Vitamin D and risk of multiple sclerosis: A Mendelian Randomization Study. PLoS Medicine. 2015;**12**: e1001866

[64] Gianfrancesco MA, Glymour MM, Walter S, et al. Causal effect of genetic variants associated with body mass index on multiple sclerosis susceptibility. American Journal of Epidemiology. 2017;**185**:162-171

[65] Handunnetthi L, Ramagopalan SV, Ebers GC. Multiple sclerosis, vitamin

D, and HLA-DRB1*15. Neurology. 2010;**74**:1905-1910

[66] Sandberg L, Biström M, Salzer J, et al. Vitamin D and axonal injury in multiple sclerosis. Multiple Sclerosis. 2016;**22**:1027-1031

[67] Ascherio A, Munger KL, White R, et al. Vitamin D as an early predictor of multiple sclerosis activity and progression. JAMA Neurology. 2014;**71**:306-314

[68] Fitzgerald KC, Munger KL, Köchert K, et al. Association of Vitamin D levels with multiple sclerosis activity and progression in patients receiving interferon beta-1b. JAMA Neurology. 2015;**72**:1458-1465

[69] Heydarpour P, Amini H, Khoshkish S, et al. Potential impact of air pollution on multiple sclerosis in Tehran, Iran. Neuroepidemiology. 2014;**43**:233-238

[70] Chen H, Kwong JC, Copes R, et al. Living near major roads and the incidence of dementia, Parkinson's disease, and multiple sclerosis: A population-based cohort study. Lancet. 2017;**389**:718-726

[71] Palacios N, Munger KL, Fitzgerald KC, et al. Exposure to particulate matter air pollution and risk of multiple sclerosis in two large cohorts of US nurses. Environment International. 2017;**109**:64-72

[72] Jeanjean M, Bind M-A, Roux J, et al. Ozone, NO2 and PM10 are associated with the occurrence of multiple sclerosis relapses. Evidence from seasonal multi-pollutant analyses. Environmental Research. 2018;**163**:43-52

[73] Handel AE, Williamson AJ, Disanto G, et al. Smoking and multiple sclerosis: An updated meta-analysis. PLoS One. 2011;**6**:e16149

[74] Hawkes CH. Smoking is a risk factor for multiple sclerosis: A metanalysis. Multiple Sclerosis. 2007;**13**:610-615

[75] Hedström AK, Bäärnhielm M, Olsson T, et al. Tobacco smoking, but not Swedish snuff use, increases the risk of multiple sclerosis. Neurology. 2009;**73**:696-701

[76] Hedström AK, Hillert J, Olsson T, et al. Smoking and multiple sclerosis susceptibility. European Journal of Epidemiology. 2013;**28**:867-874

[77] Poorolajal J, Bahrami M, Karami M, et al. Effect of smoking on multiple sclerosis: A meta-analysis. Journal of Public Health (Oxford, England). 2017;**39**:312-320

[78] Hedström AK, Olsson T, Alfredsson L. Smoking is a major preventable risk factor for multiple sclerosis. Multiple Sclerosis. 2016;**22**:1021-1026

[79] Ghadirian P, Dadgostar B, Azani R, et al. A case-control study of the association between socio-demographic, lifestyle and medical history factors and multiple sclerosis. Canadian Journal of Public Health. 2001;**92**:281-285

[80] Salzer J, Hallmans G, Nyström M, et al. Smoking as a risk factor for multiple sclerosis. Multiple Sclerosis. 2013;**19**:1022-1027

[81] Abdollahpour I, Nedjat S, Sahraian MA, et al. Waterpipe smoking associated with multiple sclerosis: A population-based incident case-control study. Multiple Sclerosis. 2017;**23**:1328-1335

[82] Mikaeloff Y, Caridade G, Tardieu M, et al. Parental smoking at home and the risk of childhood-onset multiple sclerosis in children. Brain. 2007;**130**:2589-2595

[83] Lavery AM, Collins BN, Waldman AT, et al. The contribution of secondhand tobacco smoke exposure to pediatric multiple sclerosis risk. Multiple Sclerosis. 2019;**25**:515-522

[84] Hedström AK, Bäärnhielm M, Olsson T, et al. Exposure to environmental tobacco smoke is associated with increased risk for multiple sclerosis. Multiple Sclerosis. 2011;**17**:788-793

[85] Hedström AK, Alfredsson L, Lundkvist Ryner M, et al. Smokers run increased risk of developing anti-natalizumab antibodies. Multiple Sclerosis. 2014;**20**:1081-1085

[86] Hedström AK, Ryner M, Fink K, et al. Smoking and risk of treatment-induced neutralizing antibodies to interferon β-1a. Multiple Sclerosis. 2014;**20**:445-450

[87] Hedström AK, Hillert J, Olsson T, et al. Nicotine might have a protective effect in the etiology of multiple sclerosis. Multiple Sclerosis. 2013;**19**:1009-1013

[88] Nizri E, Irony-Tur-Sinai M, Lory O, et al. Activation of the cholinergic anti-inflammatory system by nicotine attenuates neuroinflammation via suppression of Th1 and Th17 responses. Journal of Immunology. 2009;**183**:6681-6688

[89] Hedström AK, Katsoulis M, Hössjer O, et al. The interaction between smoking and HLA genes in multiple sclerosis: Replication and refinement. European Journal of Epidemiology. 2017;**32**:909-919

[90] Briggs FBS, Acuna B, Shen L, et al. Smoking and risk of multiple sclerosis: Evidence of modification by NAT1 variants. Epidemiology. 2014;**25**:605-614

[91] Munger KL, Bentzen J, Laursen B, et al. Childhood body mass index and multiple sclerosis risk: A long-term cohort study. Multiple Sclerosis. 2013;**19**:1323-1329

[92] Langer-Gould A, Brara SM, Beaber BE, et al. Childhood obesity and risk of pediatric multiple sclerosis and clinically isolated syndrome. Neurology. 2013;**80**:548-552

[93] Hedström AK, Olsson T, Alfredsson L. Body mass index during adolescence, rather than childhood, is critical in determining MS risk. Multiple Sclerosis. 2016;**22**:878-883

[94] Wesnes K, Riise T, Casetta I, et al. Body size and the risk of multiple sclerosis in Norway and Italy: The EnvIMS study. Multiple Sclerosis. 2015;**21**:388-395

[95] Mokry LE, Ross S, Timpson NJ, et al. Obesity and multiple sclerosis: A Mendelian Randomization Study. PLoS Medicine. 2016;**13**:e1002053

[96] Procaccini C, Pucino V, Mantzoros CS, et al. Leptin in autoimmune diseases. Metabolism. 2015;**64**:92-104

[97] Lumeng CN, Bodzin JL, Saltiel AR. Obesity induces a phenotypic switch in adipose tissue macrophage polarization. The Journal of Clinical Investigation. 2007;**117**:175-184

[98] Matarese G, Carrieri PB, La Cava A, et al. Leptin increase in multiple sclerosis associates with reduced number of CD4(+)CD25+ regulatory T cells. Proceedings of the National Academy of Sciences of the United States of America. 2005;**102**:5150-5155

[99] Matarese G, Carrieri PB, Montella S, et al. Leptin as a metabolic link to multiple sclerosis. Nature Reviews: Neurology. 2010;**6**:455-461

[100] Wortsman J, Matsuoka LY, Chen TC, et al. Decreased bioavailability of vitamin D in obesity. The American Journal of Clinical Nutrition. 2000;**72**:690-693

[101] Hedström AK, Lima Bomfim I, Hillert J, et al. Obesity interacts with infectious mononucleosis in risk of multiple sclerosis. European Journal of Neurology. 2015;**22**:578-e38

[102] Karlsson EA, Beck MA. The burden of obesity on infectious disease. Experimental Biology and Medicine (Maywood, N.J.). 2010;**235**:1412-1424

[103] Paich HA, Sheridan PA, Handy J, et al. Overweight and obese adult humans have a defective cellular immune response to pandemic H1N1 influenza A virus. Obesity (Silver Spring). 2013;**21**:2377-2386

[104] Hedström AK, Hillert J, Olsson T, et al. Alcohol as a modifiable lifestyle factor affecting multiple sclerosis risk. JAMA Neurology. 2014;**71**:300-305

[105] Imhof A, Froehlich M, Brenner H, et al. Effect of alcohol consumption on systemic markers of inflammation. Lancet. 2001;**357**:763-767

[106] Pasala S, Barr T, Messaoudi I. Impact of alcohol abuse on the adaptive immune system. Alcohol Research: Current Reviews. 2015;**37**:185-197

[107] Romeo J, Wärnberg J, Nova E, et al. Moderate alcohol consumption and the immune system: A review. The British Journal of Nutrition. 2007;**98**(Suppl. 1):S111-S115

[108] Hedström AK, Olsson T, Alfredsson L. The increased risk of multiple sclerosis associated with HLA-DRB1*15:01 and smoking is modified by alcohol consumption. Scientific Reports. 2021;**11**:21237

[109] Azizov V, Dietel K, Steffen F, et al. Ethanol consumption inhibits TFH cell responses and the development of autoimmune arthritis. Nature Communications. 2020;**11**:1998

[110] Ghalamfarsa G, Mahmoudi M, Mohammadnia-Afrouzi M, et al. IL-21 and IL-21 receptor in the immunopathogenesis of multiple sclerosis. Journal of Immunotoxicology. 2016;**13**:274-285

[111] Gharibi T, Hosseini A, Marofi F, et al. IL-21 and IL-21-producing T cells are involved in multiple sclerosis severity and progression. Immunology Letters. 2019;**216**:12-20

[112] Barbhaiya M, Costenbader KH. Environmental exposures and the development of systemic lupus erythematosus. Current Opinion in Rheumatology. 2016;**28**:497-505

[113] Carlé A, Bülow Pedersen I, Knudsen N, et al. Graves' hyperthyroidism and moderate alcohol consumption: Evidence for disease prevention. Clinical Endocrinology. 2013;**79**:111-119

[114] Carlé A, Pedersen IB, Knudsen N, et al. Moderate alcohol consumption may protect against overt autoimmune hypothyroidism: A population-based case-control study. European Journal of Endocrinology. 2012;**167**:483-490

[115] Andersen C, Søndergaard HB, Bang Oturai D, et al. Alcohol consumption in adolescence is associated with a lower risk of multiple sclerosis in a Danish cohort. Multiple Sclerosis. 2019;**25**:1572-1579

[116] Hedström AK, Mowry EM, Gianfrancesco MA, et al. High consumption of coffee is associated with decreased multiple sclerosis risk; results from two independent studies.

Journal of Neurology, Neurosurgery, and Psychiatry. 2016;**87**:454-460

[117] Tola MR, Granieri E, Malagù S, et al. Dietary habits and multiple sclerosis. A retrospective study in Ferrara, Italy. Acta Neurol (Napoli). 1994;**16**:189-197

[118] Millen BE, Abrams S, Adams-Campbell L, Anderson CA, Brenna JT, Campbell WW, et al. The 2015 dietary guidelines advisory committee scientific report: Development and major conclusions. Advances in Nutrition. 16 May 2016;7(3):438-444. DOI: 10.3945/an.116.012120. PMID: 27184271; PMCID: PMC4863277

[119] Tsutsui S, Schnermann J, Noorbakhsh F, et al. A1 adenosine receptor upregulation and activation attenuates neuroinflammation and demyelination in a model of multiple sclerosis. The Journal of Neuroscience. 2004;**24**:1521-1529

[120] Chen GQ, Chen YY, Wang XS, et al. Chronic caffeine treatment attenuates experimental autoimmune encephalomyelitis induced by guinea pig spinal cord homogenates in Wistar rats. Brain Research. 2010;**1309**:116-125

[121] Chen X, Ghribi O, Geiger JD. Caffeine protects against disruptions of the blood-brain barrier in animal models of Alzheimer's and Parkinson's diseases. Journal of Alzheimer's Disease. 2010;**20**(Suppl. 1):S127-S141

[122] D'hooghe MB, Haentjens P, Nagels G, et al. Alcohol, coffee, fish, smoking and disease progression in multiple sclerosis. European Journal of Neurology. 2012;**19**:616-624

[123] Krementsov DN, Case LK, Hickey WF, et al. Exacerbation of autoimmune neuroinflammation by dietary sodium is genetically controlled and sex specific. The FASEB Journal. 2015;**29**:3446-3457

[124] Kleinewietfeld M, Manzel A, Titze J, et al. Sodium chloride drives autoimmune disease by the induction of pathogenic TH17 cells. Nature. 2013;**496**:518-522

[125] Hucke S, Eschborn M, Liebmann M, et al. Sodium chloride promotes pro-inflammatory macrophage polarization thereby aggravating CNS autoimmunity. Journal of Autoimmunity. 2016;**67**:90-101

[126] Cortese M, Yuan C, Chitnis T, et al. No association between dietary sodium intake and the risk of multiple sclerosis. Neurology. 2017;**89**:1322-1329

[127] McDonald J, Graves J, Waldman A, et al. A case-control study of dietary salt intake in pediatric-onset multiple sclerosis. Multiple Sclerosis and Related Disorders. 2016;**6**:87-92

[128] Farez MF, Fiol MP, Gaitán MI, et al. Sodium intake is associated with increased disease activity in multiple sclerosis. Journal of Neurology, Neurosurgery, and Psychiatry. 2015;**86**:26-31

[129] Fitzgerald KC, Munger KL, Hartung H-P, et al. Sodium intake and multiple sclerosis activity and progression in BENEFIT. Annals of Neurology. 2017;**82**:20-29

[130] Nourbakhsh B, Graves J, Casper TC, et al. Dietary salt intake and time to relapse in paediatric multiple sclerosis. Journal of Neurology, Neurosurgery, and Psychiatry. 2016;**87**:1350-1353

[131] Bjørnevik K, Chitnis T, Ascherio A, et al. Polyunsaturated fatty acids and the risk of multiple sclerosis. Multiple Sclerosis. 2017;**23**:1830-1838

[132] Hoare S, Lithander F, van der Mei I, et al. Higher intake of omega-3 polyunsaturated fatty acids is associated with a decreased risk of a first clinical diagnosis of central nervous system demyelination: Results from the Ausimmune Study. Multiple Sclerosis. 2016;**22**:884-892

[133] Yadav V, Marracci G, Kim E, et al. Low-fat, plant-based diet in multiple sclerosis: A randomized controlled trial. Multiple Sclerosis and Related Disorders. 2016;**9**:80-90

[134] Kouchaki E, Afarini M, Abolhassani J, et al. High-dose ω-3 fatty acid plus Vitamin D3 supplementation affects clinical symptoms and metabolic status of patients with multiple sclerosis: A Randomized Controlled Clinical Trial. The Journal of Nutrition. 2018;**148**:1380-1386

[135] Azary S, Schreiner T, Graves J, et al. Contribution of dietary intake to relapse rate in early paediatric multiple sclerosis. Journal of Neurology, Neurosurgery, and Psychiatry. 2018;**89**:28-33

[136] Timmermans S, Bogie JFJ, Vanmierlo T, et al. High fat diet exacerbates neuroinflammation in an animal model of multiple sclerosis by activation of the Renin Angiotensin system. Journal of Neuroimmune Pharmacology. 2014;**9**:209-217

[137] Uranga RM, Bruce-Keller AJ, Morrison CD, et al. Intersection between metabolic dysfunction, high fat diet consumption, and brain aging. Journal of Neurochemistry. 2010;**114**:344-361

[138] Jakimovski D, Guan Y, Ramanathan M, et al. Lifestyle-based modifiable risk factors in multiple sclerosis: Review of experimental and clinical findings. Neurodegenerative Disease Management. 2019;**9**:149-172

[139] Hedström AK, Åkerstedt T, Hillert J, et al. Shift work at young age is associated with increased risk for multiple sclerosis. Annals of Neurology. 2011;**70**:733-741

[140] Hedström AK, Åkerstedt T, Olsson T, et al. Shift work influences multiple sclerosis risk. Multiple Sclerosis. 2015;**21**:1195-1199

[141] Gustavsen S, Søndergaard HB, Oturai DB, et al. Shift work at young age is associated with increased risk of multiple sclerosis in a Danish population. Multiple Sclerosis and Related Disorders. 2016;**9**:104-109

[142] Farez MF, Mascanfroni ID, Méndez-Huergo SP, et al. Melatonin Contributes to the Seasonality of Multiple Sclerosis Relapses. Cell. 2015;**162**:1338-1352

[143] Fan Y, Zhang J. Dietary modulation of intestinal microbiota: Future opportunities in experimental autoimmune encephalomyelitis and multiple sclerosis. Frontiers in Microbiology. 16 Apr 2019;**10**:740. DOI: 10.3389/fmicb.2019.00740. PMID: 31040833; PMCID: PMC6476896

[144] Schepici G, Silvestro S, Bramanti P, et al. The gut microbiota in multiple sclerosis: An overview of clinical trials. Cell Transplantation. 2019;**28**:1507-1527

[145] Calvo-Barreiro L, Eixarch H, Montalban X, et al. Combined therapies to treat complex diseases: The role of the gut microbiota in multiple sclerosis. Autoimmunity Reviews. 2018;**17**:165-174

Section 3

Research into Optical Neuroimaging in Multiple Sclerosis

Chapter 4

Optical Coherence Tomography (OCT) and Angio-OCT Imaging Techniques in Multiple Sclerosis Patients with or without Optic Neuritis

Bilyana Mihaylova and Sylvia Cherninkova

Abstract

The visual system is typically affected in multiple sclerosis (MS) patients. The most common ocular manifestation during the clinical course of the disease is optic neuritis (ON). Optical coherence tomography (OCT) is well-established tool for biomedical imaging that enables detection of retinal nerve fiber layer and ganglion cell layer thickness reduction – biomarkers of axonal damage and neuronal loss in MS. And OCT angiography (angio-OCT) is another imaging method for assessing retinal and choroidal vessels with no need of contrast dye injection. In our prospective study, we investigate parafoveal and peripapillary microvascular retinal networks in 18 MS patients (35 eyes) through angio-OCT (AngioVue, OptoVue). According to our results, early structural changes in MS patients without previous history of acute ON episode are unable to be detected. As a follow-up imaging technique, OCT is very useful for changes in axonal thickness and defines the progression rate of the disease. Angio-OCT vis-à-vis OCT investigation detects the ocular perfusion reduction before the appearance of structural changes. From all investigated structural and density parameters only those in superficial capillary plexus show significant changes in MS patients without ON. For accurate diagnostic and following-up process, both structural and vascular parameters need to be assessed in MS patients.

Keywords: multiple sclerosis, optical coherence tomography, angio-OCT, vessel density, RNFL, GCC

1. Introduction

Multiple sclerosis (MS) is a chronic autoimmune inflammatory demyelinating disease of the central nervous system that is accompanied by a parallel process of neurodegeneration (axonal and neuronal), and subsequent atrophy of the brain and spinal cord. The impairment of the visual sensory pathways and more specifically of the optic nerves is a common clinically manifested finding in MS patients at various stages (at onset or a later stage) of the disease. Optic neuritis (ON), in the majority of MS patients, is characterized by a significant improvement or even complete recovery of the visual functions, however, advanced neuroophthalmological studies, that include automated (computerized) threshold static perimetry, color vision testing, contrast sensitivity examination, etc., demonstrate discrete or more pronounced residual symptoms. Loss of retinal ganglion cells (GCL) and optic nerve atrophy, in combination with signs of inflammation, are established in postmortem studies of eye structures of MS patients [1–3]. Over the last 10–15 years, optical coherence tomography (OCT) has been assessed as a highly sensitive and informative technique to follow up the process of neurodegeneration in MS. The method is characterized by high definition and allows for studying individual retinal layers – their morphology and thickness measured in microns (μm).

2. Neuro-ophthalmological manifestations in MS patients

Neuro-ophthalmological manifestations in MS include visual pathways lesions, oculomotor dysfunctions, pupillary disorders, and other ocular impairments.

As the first (monosymptomatic) disorder in MS, ON is the most frequent ocular manifestation (up to 25% of cases) [4]. During the clinical course of the disease 30–70% of all MS patients develop ON [5, 6]. The following features are observed: decreased visual acuity, visual field defects, color vision disturbances, pupillary disorders, retro-ocular or orbital pain, positive visual phenomena, optic nerve head (ONH) changes, and Uhthoff's sign. In most cases, it occurs as retrobulbar neuritis, but also it could be observed as papillitis (mild or severe edema; local or diffuse edema; with or without ONH or retinal hemorrhages). In the acute ON phase, almost all MS patients have decreased contrast sensitivity using Pelli-Robson's table [7].

In MS patients with established unilateral ON, and no previous history of such, could be observed variations in visual functions of the contralateral eye, which are: mild visual field defects, impairment of contrast sensitivity and color vision, relative afferent pupillary defect (RAPD), and partial atrophy of the optic nerve.

According to the Optic Neuritis Treatment Trial (ONTT), the visual acuity during ON could vary in wide ranges: from 1.0 (Decimal acuity) to counting fingers in front of the eye, hand movement, light perception, or lack of the light perception [8]. ON acute phase is possible to be followed by a period of visual functions deficit: decreased visual acuity (6 months – 1 year); visual field defects (6 months); abnormal color vision (6 months); decreased contrast sensitivity with Pelli-Robson's table (6 months); and RAPD (6 months).

Visual field defects include the following options: central and cecocentral scotomas, arcuate and altitudinal defects, diffuse loss of retinal light sensitivity in central 30°, chiasmal defects, retrochiasmal defects, and other visual field defects [7].

Oculomotor disorders in MS are results of demyelinating lesions in infranuclear, nuclear, supranuclear, and internuclear structures. In 15% of MS patients, ocular disorders are clinical onset debut of the disease and could precede months or years of the appearance of other neurological features. The most common infranuclear lesion is those of n. abducens (CN VI), less common is those of n. oculomotorius (CN III), and least common is those of n. trochlearis (CN IV) [9]. Internuclear ophthalmoparesis (INO) is a result of fasciculus longitudinalis medialis demyelinating lesions between nuclei of n. oculomotorius and n. abducens. The nerve impulse transmission along a neuron pathway is impaired, and clinically it is manifested as a lack of or partially limited adduction in the ipsilateral eye [10]. In the literature, there is a rule: the most common reason for bilateral INO in young adults and adults is MS [6]. Combinations of oculomotor lesions such as one-and-a-half syndrome describe horizontal eye movement disorder – ipsilateral conjugate horizontal gaze palsy (one) and ipsilateral INO (a half).

Pupillary abnormalities are not uncommon in MS [11]. According to different authors, they seem to be underestimated independently of the presence of ON [12]. The following disturbances in pupillary reactions have been reported: 1. RAPD during the acute ON phase. It could be seen even after full visual functions recovery; 2. Ophthalmoparesis oculomotoria interna a rare pathological pupillary manifestation, which is caused by n. oculomotorius infranuclear lesions and concomitant parasympathetic nerve fibers damage; 3. Argyll-Robertson's syndrome rarely has been evaluated in MS; 4. Horner's syndrome; and 5. Pupillary hippus.

Other ocular manifestations in MS, which could be observed are 1. Peripheral retinal periphlebitis – a vasculitis that affects approximately 10% of patients with MS and is associated with higher disease activity in relapses [13]; 2. Microcystic macular edema in 0.5–5% of patients with MS and is associated probably with MS activity or previous ON [13]; and 3. Uveitis – it is an intraocular inflammation of the uvea, retina, or vitreous body and appears rarely in MS. The association of MS with uveitis is unclear. The most common type of uveitis seems to be intermediate uveitis, which primarily involves vitreous, peripheral retina, and pars plana of the ciliary body. Another type that could be observed in MS is granulomatous anterior uveitis [14].

2.1 Optical coherence tomography as an imaging method in ophthalmology

OCT is a relatively new noninvasive imaging technology that uses near-infrared light to generate high-resolution, cross-sectional, or three-dimensional images of the eye [15]. It was demonstrated in 1991 by David Huang. Then he established for the first time the applicability of the low-coherence interferometry in the quantitative assessment of biological systems. The technique was initially applied for imaging in the eye. Up to now, OCT has had the largest clinical impact in ophthalmology. OCT has revolutionized the clinical practice of ophthalmology and become a standard of clinical care for diagnosis, treatment, and monitoring of many posterior segment diseases [15]. With a longitudinal resolution of 5–7 μm OCT provides images comparable and close to an in-vivo "optical biopsy" of the retina.

OCT uses the light from a broadband light source, which is divided into a reference and a sample beam. The sample beam backscatters from the retina and interferes with the reference beam. This interference pattern is used to measure the light echoes versus the depth profile of the tissue in vivo [16, 17].

OCT is used extensively for analyzing the morphology and quantitative changes of retinal layer volume and thickness of the posterior segment structures such as macula, GCL, ONH, retinal nerve fiber layer (RNFL), and choroidea. Anterior segment-OCT (AS-OCT) is used basically for visualizing cornea and corneal thickness, anterior chamber angle, iris, irido-corneal apposition, etc. [18].

Currently available are different OCT technologies, namely time domain (TD-OCT), spectral domain (SD-OCT), swept-source (SS-OCT) technology, and others that are in development [19, 20]. The measurements with different OCT devices show significant differences from one instrument to another, therefore, the providing values are noninterchangeable in healthy eyes and in MS patients, even when the comparisons are between SD-OCT and TD-OCT devices or only between two different SD-OCT devices [21–23].

The next two figures (**Figures 1** and **2**) represent the most important structural information in the retina obtained with OCT concerning MS patients. In **Figure 1** is shown *ONH/GCC* (ganglion cell complex) *OU* (oculus uterque – Latin for both eyes) *Report* image obtained with angio-OCT (AngioVue, OptoVue) in a healthy woman. *GCC NBD* (Normative Database) *Reference* and *GCC Analysis* give a summary of

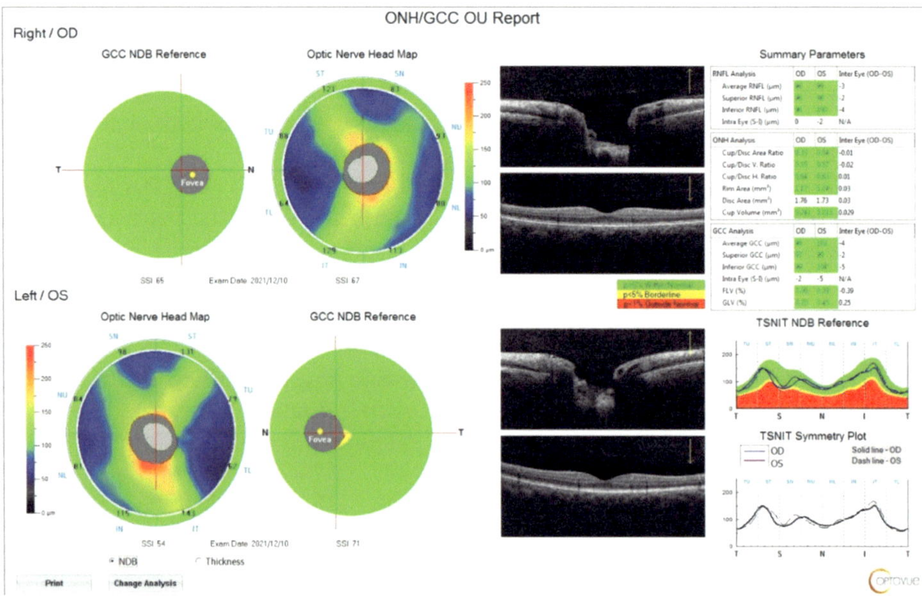

Figure 1.
ONH/GCC OU Report (AngioVue, OptoVue) in a healthy woman.

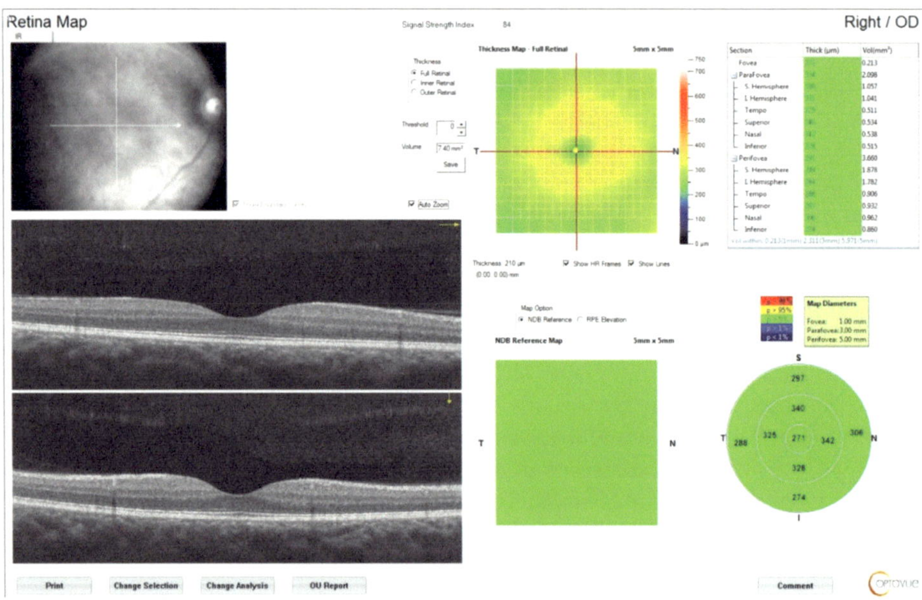

Figure 2.
Retina map report of right eye in a healthy woman.

inner retinal layers thickness in macular area (bodies + dendrites + axons of ganglion cells). *Optic Nerve Head Map*, *RNFL Analysis*, and *ONH Analysis* provide information about ONH parameters (vertical and horizontal cup/disc area ratio, disc/rim area, and cup volume) and RNFL thickness around ONH (Average/Superior Half/Inferior Half /and combinations). Through color codes, the protocol also provides quantitative data, with which retinal layer thickness could be interpreted. Green color means normal thickness compared to NDB, yellow color is borderline thickness, and red color is significantly reduced thickness. TSNIT NDB Reference shows RNFL thickness curve in fourth peripapillary quadrants according to the ISNT rule – the RNFL thickness decreases as follows – inferior quadrant (I) → superior quadrant (S) → nasal quadrant (N) → temporal quadrant (T). The part *TSNIT Symmetry Plot* shows RNFL thickness symmetry between both eyes.

In **Figure 2** could be seen *Retina Map Report* obtained with angio-OCT (AngioVue, OptoVue) in a healthy woman. Except infrared image of the eye fundus, OCT B-scan in macular zone central through the fovea, the protocol gives information about retinal thickness in macular area. The examiner has the possibilities to choose what thickness to analyze – full retinal/inner retinal/outer retinal or all of them if needed. In the same way as pervious protocol, the information about retinal thickness could be interpreted by colors and values compared with reference data.

2.2 Optical coherence tomography as a window to the MS brain

Over the last 10–15 years, OCT has been assessed as a highly sensitive and informative technique to investigate retinal neuro-axonal loss and follow up on the process of neurodegeneration in MS [24]. Using OCT, we can directly examine a structure in the central nervous system (CNS), such as the retina, which consists of isolated axons, because as part of the RNFL they are not myelinated. The assessment of the GCL thickness, which consists of the three innermost layers of the retina (axons + bodies + dendrites of the ganglion cells) in the macular area, provides information on the neuro-axonal loss. Also, the reduction in peripapillary RNFL (pRNFL) thickness has been reported in different MS-related subtypes as an expression of the axonal loss. Multiple studies show a significant decrease in RNFL thickness in MS patients who have had ON, in comparison to a healthy control group or fellow eye that is not affected by ON [25–32]. A more manifest thinning of RNFL is seen in the temporal axons of the retina, due to the predilection impairment of the papillomacular bundle by the inflammatory process. Studies using OCT method in MS patients with no history of optic neuritis and completely normal visual functions also demonstrate a reduction in RNFL thickness, but to a lower extent compared to the eyes affected by optic neuritis [25, 28, 33–35]. This difference is a result of the more severe axonal loss in the retina in eyes with history of ON. Even in the absence of previous ON episodes, RNFL reduction may occur as a biomarker of disease progression [36].

In 2017 a meta-analysis proposes OCT scans in two different ocular regions – ONH and macular area to be routinely included in MS clinical practice because OCT could have the role of a predictive biomarker in disease duration and clinical assessment [32].

Figures 3 and **4** are examples of the same protocols as the previous two pictures but provide information about structural retinal changes in young MS patients (25 years) investigated 6 months after an acute ON episode of the right eye. The significantly reduced RNFL, GCC thickness, and total retinal thickness in the affected eye are obvious. What makes an impression is also the affected retinal structures (total retinal thickness, blue color code) of the fellow (left) eye with no history of acute ON episode.

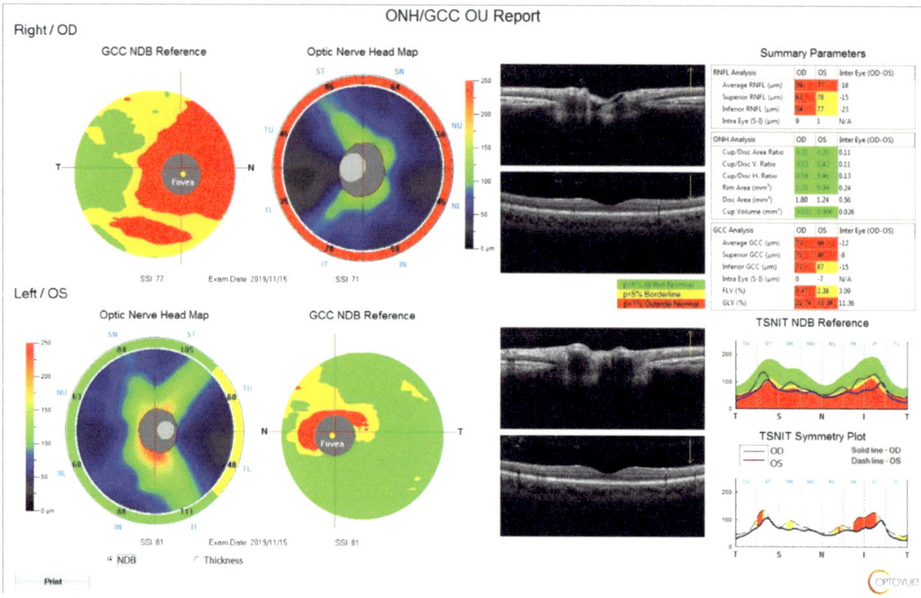

Figure 3.
ONH/GCC OU Report of a young male patient (25 years) after an acute episode of MS associated ON in right eye.

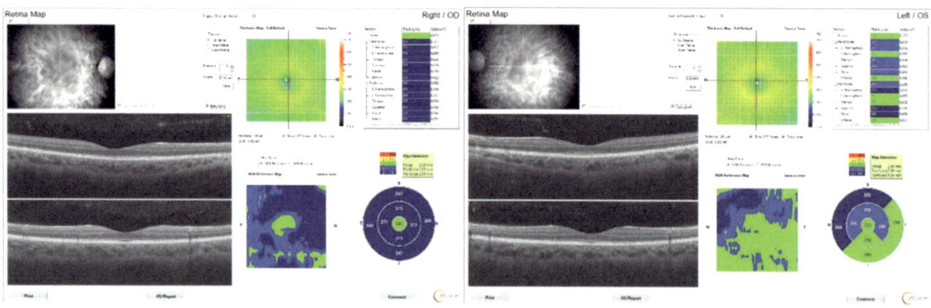

Figure 4.
Retina Map OD/OS Report of a young male patient (25 years) after an acute episode of MS associated ON in right eye.

2.3 OCT-angiography in MS patients

Frequent association between neuronal changes in MS and vascular diseases is mentioned in different publications, although past reports show controversial results. These vascular changes can possibly contribute to neuronal or degenerative dysfunction in patients with MS [37].

The entry into the clinic of OCT-angiography (angio-OCT) gives new expectations for better knowledge and understanding of retinal and neurodegenerative diseases [38]. Angio-OCT is an imaging method for assessing retinal and choroidal vessels with no need of contrast dye injection. It images blood flow due to red blood cells movement and changes in reflectivity signals after a series of A-scans at one particular point [39]. The areas in ocular fundus, which are constant and no movement is detected there, show no change in reflectivity signals, but those once with moving objects show large deviations in reflectivity signals. In the retina, there are no changeable areas giving differences in reflectivity signals with the exception of blood vessels. And while with the fluorescein angiography imaging method only superficial retinal vessels are visualized, with angio-OCT all retinal capillary networks are visualized, including the choroidal capillary layer [40].

This new imaging method assesses retinal vessel density parameters in both areas – macula and ONH. Some recent reports present convincing and detailed data that significant vascular abnormalities are involved in MS pathology. A vessel density reduction in eyes of MS patients is available when compared to controls [38]. Some papers reporting the above-mentioned statements suggest that angio-OCT could be a good marker of disease and disability in MS [41].

In **Figure 5a** is shown the very informative *Angio Retina QuickVue Report* of the right eye (macular area) in a healthy woman. The four angio images at the top of the picture represent from left to right, respectively, superficial capillary plexus (from inner limiting membrane – ILM to inner plexiform layer – IPL), deep capillary plexus

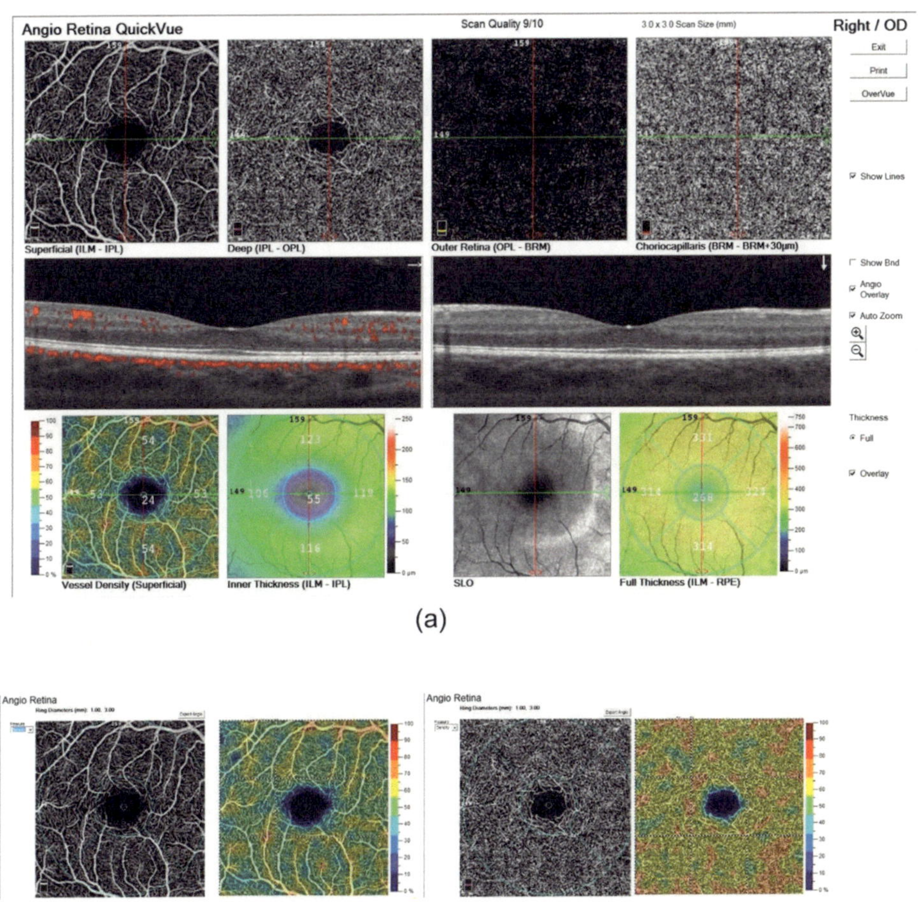

Figure 5.
a. Angio Retina QuickVue Report of the right eye (macular area) in a healthy woman. b. Part of Angio Retina Report in healthy woman showing differences in angio images and color codes of superficial (both left images) and deep capillary plexus density.

(from IPL to outer plexiform layer – OPL), outer retina (from OPL to Bruch's membrane – BRM), and choriocapillaris (from BRM + 30 μm). Quantitative values are also represented for superficial vessel density and inner and full retinal thickness. 5B part shows differences in angio images and color codes of superficial (both left images) and deep capillary plexus density.

Figure 6 best illustrates vessel density of the peripapillary capillary plexus through *Angio Disc QuickVue Vessel Report*. In addition to data about peripapillary vessel density parameters, the report also provides such about pRNFL thickness, ONH parameters, and angio images in different levels of the peripapillary area.

Figure 7 is an example of *Angio Retina QuickVue Report* of a young male patient (25 years) after acute episode of MS associated ON in right eye. Easily can be observed the difference in superficial vessel density between the healthy subject (**Figure 5a** and **b** in superficial capillary plexus) and the patient with history of ON – diffuse and local vessel density reduction are observed in this example.

Figure 7 is an example of *Angio Disc QuickVue Report* in an MS patient (46 years, male) who demonstrated significantly reduced vessel density of peripapillary capillary plexus after two ON episodes of the left eye. The difference in reduced vessel density (local and diffuse) can be easily observed when **Figures 6** and **7** are compared not only by reduced density values but also by color codes (blue for reduced density) and angio RPC images (RPC – radial peripapillary capillary).

2.4 Our experience

In our prospective randomized study, 38 participants were included – 18 patients with confirmed MS (35 eyes) and 20 healthy volunteers (20 eyes). The research was conducted over a year (2020–2021) at two different hospitals – 1) Clinic of Nervous Diseases at University Hospital "Alexandrovska" in Sofia, Bulgaria where the MS diagnostic tests and

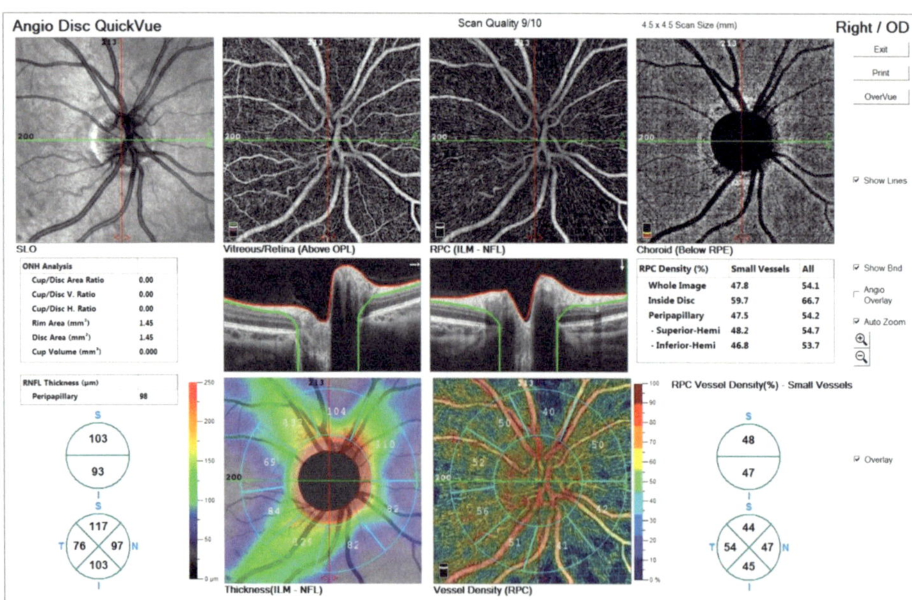

Figure 6.
Angio Disc QuickVue Report showing vessel density of the peripapillary capillary plexus in a healthy woman.

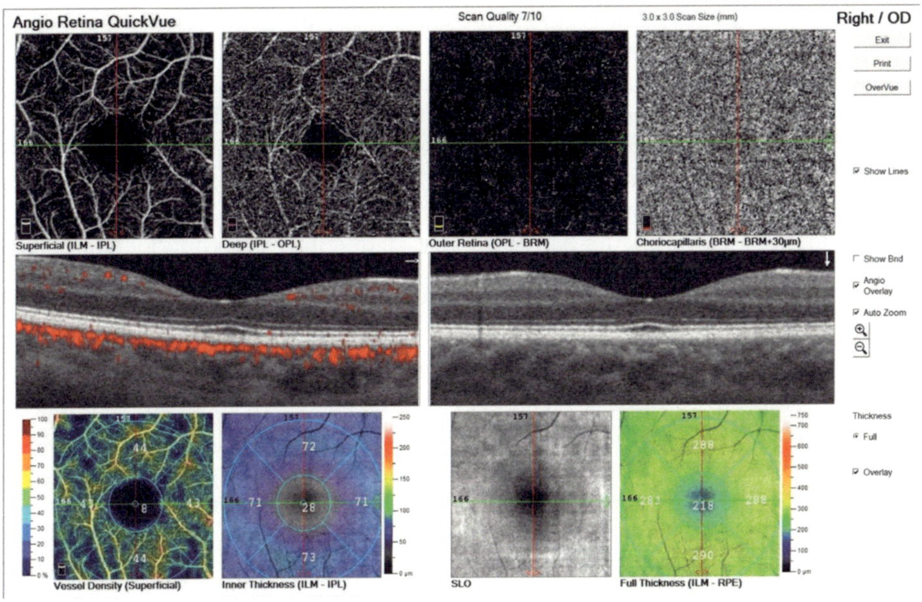

Figure 7.
Angio Retina QuickVue Report of a young male patient (25 years) after acute episode of MS associated ON in right eye.

neurologic following-up are performed and 2) Eye Hospital "Vision" in Sofia, Bulgaria where complete eye examination, specialized ophthalmology tests, and imaging methods (OCT and angio-OCT) are performed. All subjects included in this work gave their consent for inclusion before they participated. The work was conducted in accordance with the Declaration of Helsinki. The authors have no relevant financial or nonfinancial conflicts of interest to declare. The purpose of our work is to investigate parafoveal and peripapillary microvascular retinal networks through angio-OCT (AngioVue, OptoVue).

The MS patients were divided into two groups: 1. MS with previous episodes of ON (19 eyes) and 2. MS without previous episodes of ON (16 eyes). All subjects underwent the standard set of neuro-ophthalmologic examination. In addition, angio-OCT was performed – structural (pRNFL and GCC) and vessel density (Superficial / Deep in macular area and RPC) parameters were achieved for each single (see theoretical part and methodology – Sections 2.1; 2.2; and 2.3 for used AngioVue protocols).

The statistical analysis includes descriptive statistics – results are represented as a mean and standard deviation (Mean±SD); one-sample Kolmogorov-Smirnov test – to check the normality of distribution; Kruskal Wallis Test – nonparametric test used to determine if there are statistically significant differences between two or more independent groups in distribution different from normal; Mann-Whitney test – again nonparametric test, but it is used to determine if there is statistically significant difference between two independent groups in distribution different from normal.

According to our results the investigation of the retinal structural parameters (GCC and pRNFL) showed:

Average pRNFL decreases in the following order: Controls (100.35 ± 8.37 µm) → MS without ON (96.44 ± 8.76 µm) → MS with ON (74.79 ± 13.28 µm). The significant difference was found between Controls and MS with ON ($p < 0.001$), and between MS with and without MS ($p < 0.001$), but such a difference was not found between Controls and MS without ON (0.265).

Average GCC decreases in the following order: Controls (96.80 ± 7.32 μm) → MS without ON (92.19 ± 5.74 μm) → MS with ON (72.89 ± 7.87 μm). The same significant differences as those in Average pRNFL were observed: between Controls and MS with ON ($p < 0.001$), and between MS with and without MS ($p < 0.001$), absence of such significance between Controls and MS without ON (0.175).

In **Table 1** is shown density (%) of the superficial capillary plexus in macular area (**Figures 5a, b** and 7). We investigated 5 density parameters: 1. Whole (Ring diameter – 3 mm) 2. Superior-Hemi (superior half of the ring) 3. Inferior-Hemi (inferior half of the ring) 4. Fovea and 5. Parafovea (Ring diameter – 1 mm). We applied a nonparametric Kruskal-Wallis statistical test for more than two independent groups. The results show that values for all 5 density parameters decrease in following order: Controls → MS without ON episode → MS with ON episode. This comparative analysis demonstrated a statistically significant difference for all 5 parameters. Therefore, another nonparametric intergroup comparative analysis was applied – Mann-Whitney test to compare two independent groups (**Table 2**). The results show a significant difference between Controls and MS with ON for all 5 density parameters. Four out of the five parameters show a significant difference between Controls and MS without ON (exception Parafovea), between the two MS groups (exception Fovea). The same statistical tests were applied to investigate the density of the deep capillary plexus (**Tables 3** and **4**).

The mean deep density values in the three groups are very close and statistical significant difference was not found with exception of one of them – Fovea. Only for this parameter additional intergroup statistical analysis was applied.

Table 4 best visualized the results after Mann-Whitney test was applied for deep density parameter – Fovea. Significantly statistical differences were detected between

Density (%) Superficial	Group	N	Mean±SD	p
1. Whole	Controls	20	49.71 ± 1.96	**<0.001**
	MS with ON	19	38.16 ± 5.47	
	MS without ON	16	47.68 ± 1.85	
2. Superior-Hemi	Controls	20	49.59 ± 2.00	**<0.001**
	MS with ON	19	38.35 ± 5.55	
	MS without ON	16	47.52 ± 1.96	
3. Inferior-Hemi	Controls	20	50.35 ± 3.77	**<0.001**
	MS with ON	19	37.95 ± 5.45	
	MS without ON	16	47.90 ± 1.87	
4. Fovea	Controls	20	23.13 ± 4.66	**<0.001**
	MS with ON	19	12.98 ± 6.68	
	MS without ON	16	13.35 ± 4.60	
5. Parafovea	Controls	20	52.62 ± 1.92	**<0.001**
	MS with ON	19	40.89 ± 5.97	
	MS without ON	16	51.39 ± 2.25	

*A p-value <**0.05** is considered to be statistically significant.*

Table 1.
Density (%) of the superficial capillary plexus. Kruskal-Wallis statistical test.

Density (%) Superficial	Comparisons		
	Controls	Controls	MS with ON
	MS with ON	MS without ON	MS without ON
	p	p	p
1. Whole	**<0.001**	**0.006**	**<0.001**
2. Superior – Hemi	**<0.001**	**0.005**	**<0.001**
3. Inferior – Hemi	**<0.001**	**0.008**	**<0.001**
4. Fovea	**<0.001**	**<0.001**	0.196
5. Parafovea	**<0.001**	0.080	**<0.001**

A p-value ***<0.05*** *is considered to be statistically significant.*

Table 2.
Density (%) of the superficial capillary plexus. Mann-Whitney statistical test.

Density (%) Deep	Group	N	Mean±SD	p
1. Whole	Controls	20	55.88 ± 2.44	0.309
	MS with ON	19	54.49 ± 3.33	
	MS without ON	16	55.71 ± 2.08	
2. Superior-Hemi	Controls	20	55.97 ± 2.42	0.389
	MS with ON	19	54.54 ± 3.46	
	MS without ON	16	55.76 ± 2.12	
3. Inferior-Hemi	Controls	20	55.79 ± 2.56	0.334
	MS with ON	19	54.43 ± 3.29	
	MS without ON	16	55.68 ± 2.19	
4. Fovea	Controls	20	39.80 ± 5.88	**<0.001**
	MS with ON	19	29.41 ± 7.73	
	MS without ON	16	30.48 ± 5.76	
5. Parafovea	Controls	20	57.56 ± 2.44	0.605
	MS with ON	19	57.17 ± 3.04	
	MS without ON	16	58.11 ± 2.24	

A p-value ***<0.05*** *is considered to be statistically significant.*

Table 3.
Density (%) of the deep capillary plexus. Kruskal-Wallis statistical test.

Controls and MS with ON/MS without ON, but that difference was not found between the two MS groups.

Table 5 illustrates the results of statistical analysis of the RPC parameters. We used represented above *Angio Disc QuickVue Report* (**Figures 6** and **8**) to provide a scanning area of 4.5×4.5 mm. The three global parameters are 1. Whole 2. Inside disc 3. Peripapillary. Mean values of 2 out of the three parameters have significant differences – Whole and Peripapillary (Kruskal-Wallis test). These two parameters were investigated additionally with Mann-Whitney test (**Table 6**). Significant differences were found between Controls and MS with ON, and between MS with and without ON.

Parameter	Comparisons		
	Controls	Controls	MS with ON
	MS with ON	MS without ON	MS without ON
	p	p	p
Fovea	**<0.001**	**<0.001**	0.446
A p-value **<0.05** *is considered to be statistically significant.*			

Table 4.
Density (%) of the deep capillary plexus. Mann-Whitney statistical test.

Angio Disc	Group	N	Mean±SD	p
1. Whole	Controls	20	50.06 ± 1.80	**<0.001**
	MS with ON	16	42.86 ± 5.98	
	MS without MS	11	50.30 ± 2.81	
2. Inside Disc	Controls	20	55.90 ± 3.98	0.216
	MS with ON	16	53.38 ± 5.64	
	MS without MS	11	53.99 ± 2.94	
3. Peripapillary	Controls	20	51.13 ± 2.53	**<0.001**
	MS with ON	16	42.26 ± 7.20	
	MS without MS	11	51.79 ± 3.64	
A p-value **<0.05** *is considered to be statistically significant.*				

Table 5.
Density (%) of the RPC plexus. Kruskal-Wallis test.

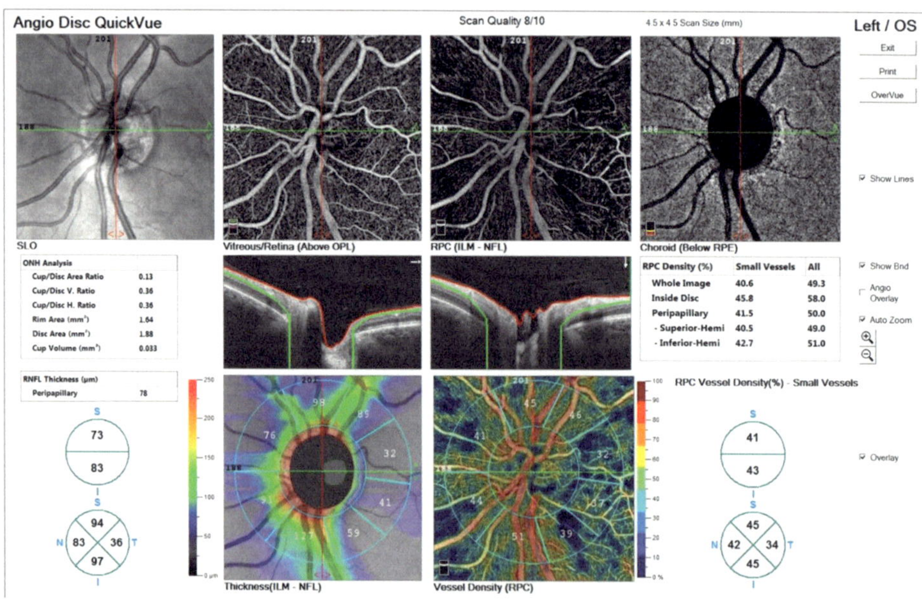

Figure 8.
Angio Disc QuickVue Report showing RPC vessel density in the patient (46 years, male) after two ON episodes of MS associated ON in left eye.

Angio Disc	Comparisons		
	Controls	Controls	MS with ON
	MS with ON	MS without ON	MS without ON
	p	P	p
Whole	**<0.001**	0.470	**<0.001**
Peripapillary	**<0.001**	0.231	**<0.001**

A p-value **<0.05** *is considered to be statistically significant.*

Table 6.
Density (%) of the RPC plexus. Mann-Whitney test.

The results show that the significant difference in Whole parameter is mainly due to density changes in peripapillary capillary vessels.

3. Conclusions

Our results could be summarized as follows: OCT (AngioVue) investigation is unable to detect significant early structural changes in global retinal thickness parameters such as Average GCC and pRNFL in MS patients without previous history of acute ON episodes. As a follow-up imaging technique, it is very useful to detect changes in the structural axonal loss. Therefore, it is especially helpful also in assessment of the disease progression rate.

The peripapillary vessel density changes, but not the whole scanned area or inside disc area, underline the significant decreases of the RPC vessel density in MS patients only with ON. Again early changes in MS without ON are not detectable in RPC.

As a whole, deep retinal microvascular network remains significantly nonaffected in MS with exception of the central macular zone (Fovea parameter), where significant decreases in vessel density could be seen independently of the disease stage (this statement is valid for both superficial and deep vessel networks). From all investigated vessel parameters, Fovea is the only one that changes significantly in both retinal networks – superficial and deep. From superficial vessel density significantly decreases as follows: Controls → MS without ON → MS with ON.

From all investigated structural and density parameters only those in superficial capillary plexus show significant changes in MS patients without ON. This particular result is of big importance in our research because it shows that vessel changes in superficial plexus precede structural changes in MS patients without ON.

In conclusion, we could summarize that angio-OCT is an important and useful imaging technique for MS patients because of its possibilities for noninvasive quantitative and qualitative evaluation of the microvascular retinal network. It is especially useful in MS patients with no previous history of acute ON episodes when significant changes in retinal microvascular network are able to be detected in the absence of significant structural changes. For accurate diagnostic and following-up process, both structural and vascular parameters need to be assessed in MS patients.

Author details

Bilyana Mihaylova[1*] and Sylvia Cherninkova[2]

1 Eye Hospital “Vision”, Sofia, Bulgaria

2 University Hospital “Alexandrovska”, Clinic of Neurology, Sofia, Bulgaria

*Address all correspondence to: b51@abv.bg

References

[1] Green A, McQuaid S, Hauser S, et al. Ocular pathology in multiple sclerosis: Retinal atrophy and inflammation irrespective of disease duration. Brain. 2010;**133**(Part 6):1591-1601

[2] Ikuta F, Zimmerman H. Distribution of plaques in seventy autopsy cases of multiple sclerosis in the United States. Neurology. 1976;**26**(6):26-28

[3] Toussaint D, Perier O, Verstappen A, et al. Clinicopathological study of the visual pathways, eyes, and cerebral hemispheres in 32 cases of disseminated sclerosis. Journal of Clinical Neuro-Ophthalmology. 1983;**3**(3):211-220

[4] Cennamo G, Romano M, Vecchio E, et al. Anatomical and functional retinal changes in multiple sclerosis. Eye (London, England). 2016;**30**(3):456-462

[5] Syc S, Saidha S, Newsome S, et al. Optical coherence tomography segmentation reveals ganglion cell layer pathology after optic neuritis. Brain. 2012;**135**(Part 2):521-533

[6] Frohman E, Frohman T, Zee D, et al. The neuro-ophthalmology of multiple sclerosis. Lancet Neurology. 2005;**4**(2):111-121

[7] Kale N. Optic neuritis as an early sign of multiple sclerosis. Eye Brain. 2016;**8**:195-202

[8] Newman N. The Optic Neuritis Treatment Trial. Ophthalmologica. 2020;**127**(4):S172-S173

[9] Bentley P, Kimber T, Schapira A. Painful third nerve palsy in MS. Neurology. 2002;**58**:1532

[10] Lavin P, Weissman B. Neuro-ophthalmology. Neurology in Clinical Practice. 1996;**1**:613-634

[11] de Seze J, Arndt C, Stojkovic T, et al. Pupillary disturbances in multiple sclerosis: Correlation with MRI findings. Journal of the Neurological Sciences. 2001;**188**:37-41

[12] Linden D, Diehl R, Berlit P. Sub-clinical autonomic disturbance in multiple sclerosis. Journal of Neurology. 1995;**242**:374-378

[13] Ortiz-Pérez S, Martínez-Lapiscina E, Gabilondo I, et al. Retinal periphlebitis is associated with multiple sclerosis severity. Neurology. 2013;**81**(10):877-881

[14] Kaya D, Kaya M, Özakbaş S, et al. Uveitis associated with multiple sclerosis: Complications and visual prognosis. International Journal of Ophthalmology. 2014;**7**(6):1010-1013

[15] Adhi M, Duker JS. Optical coherence tomography-current and future applications. Current Opinion in Ophthalmology. 2013;**24**(3):213-221

[16] Huang D, Swanson E, Lin C, et al. Optical coherence tomography. Science. 1991;**254**:1178-1181

[17] Sull A, Vuong L, Price L, et al. Comparison of spectral/Fourier domain optical coherence tomography instruments for assessment of normal macular thickness. Retina. 2010;**30**:235-245

[18] Shan J, DeBoer C, Xu BY. Anterior segment optical coherence tomography: Applications for clinical care and scientific research. Asia Pacific Journal of Ophthalmology (Phila). 2021;(323):865-9837. 2019 DOI: 10.22608/APO.201910

[19] Miller A, Roisman L, Zhang Q, et al. Comparison between spectral-domain

and swept-source optical coherence tomography angiographic imaging of choroidal neovascularization. Investigative Ophthalmology & Visual Science. 2017;**58**(3):1499-1505

[20] Davila J, Mruthyunjaya P. Updates in imaging in ocular oncology. F1000Research. 2019;**8**:1706

[21] Matlach J, Wagner M, Malzahn U, et al. Repeatability of peripapillary retinal nerve fiber layer and inner retinal thickness among two spectral domain optical coherence tomography devices. Investigative Ophthalmology & Visual Science. 2014;**55**(10):6536-6546

[22] Leite M, Rao H, Weinreb R, et al. Agreement among spectral-domain optical coherence tomography instruments for assessing retinal nerve fiber layer thickness. American Journal of Ophthalmology. 2011;**151**(1):85-92

[23] Oertel F, Zimmermann H, Brandt A, et al. Novel uses of retinal imaging with optical coherence tomography in multiple sclerosis. Expert Review of Neurotherapeutics. 2018;**27**:1-13

[24] Toosy A, Naismith R, Villoslada P. OCT as a window to the MS brain – The view becomes slightly clearer. Neurology. 2017;**89**(24):2404-2405

[25] Albrecht P, Frohlich R, Hartung H, et al. Optical coherence tomography measures axonal loss in multiple sclerosis independently of optic neuritis. Journal of Neurology. 2007;**254**(11):1595-1596

[26] Costello F, Coupland S, Hodge W, et al. Quantifying axonal loss after optic neuritis with optical coherence tomography. Annals of Neurology. 2006;**59**(6):963-999

[27] Costello F, Burton J. Retinal imaging with optical coherence tomography: A biomarker in multiple sclerosis? Eye Brain. 2018;**10**:47-63

[28] Frohman E, Dwyer M, Frohman T, et al. Relationship of optic nerve and brain conventional and non-conventional MRI measures and retinal nerve fiber layer thickness, as assessed by OCT and GDx: A pilot study. Journal of the Neurological Sciences. 2009;**282**(1-2):96-105

[29] Huang-Link Y, Fredriskson M, Link H. Benign multiple sclerosis is associated with reduced thinning of retinal nerve fiber layer and ganglion cell layers in non-optic-neuritis eyes. Journal of Clinical Neurology. 2015;**11**(3):241-247

[30] Petzold A, de Boer J, Schippling S, et al. Optical coherence tomography in multiple sclerosis: A systematic review and metaanalysis. Lancet Neurology. 2010;**9**(9):921-932

[31] Jones-Odeh E, Hammond CJ. How strong is the relationship between glaucoma, the retinal nerve fibre layer, and neurodegenerative diseases such as Alzheimer's disease and multiple sclerosis? Eye (London, England). 2015;**29**(10):1270-1284

[32] Petzold A, Balcer L, Calabresi P, et al. Retinal layer segmentation in multiple sclerosis: A systematic review and meta-analysis. Lancet Neurology. 2017;**16**(10):797-812

[33] Petzold A, Polman C, Schmidt-Erfurth U, Barkhof F. The application of optical coherence tomography to quantification of neurodegeneration in multiple sclerosis. Novartis Pharma AG, Basel, Switzerland. 2010;**68**

[34] Siger M, Dziegielewski K, Jasek L, et al. Optical coherence tomography in multiple sclerosis: Thickness of the retinal nerve fiber layer as a

potential measure of axonal loss and brain atrophy. Journal of Neurology. 2008;**255**(10):1555-1560

[35] Zaveri M, Conger A, Salter A, et al. Retinal imaging by laser polarimetry and optical coherence tomography evidence of axonal degeneration in multiple sclerosis. Archives of Neurology. 2008;**65**(7):924-928

[36] Trip S, Schlottmann P, Jones S, et al. Retinal nerve fiber layer axonal loss and visual dysfunction in optic neuritis. Annals of Neurology. 2005;**58**(3):383-391

[37] Feucht N, Maier M, Lepennetier G, et al. Optical coherence tomography angiography indicates associations of the retinal vascular network and disease activity in multiple sclerosis. Multiple Sclerosis. 2019;**25**(2):224-234

[38] Lanzillo R, Cennamo G, Criscuolo C, et al. Optical coherence tomography angiography retinal vascular network assessment in multiple sclerosis. Multiple Sclerosis Journal. 2018;**24**(13):1706-1714

[39] Borrelli E, Sadda S, Uji A, et al. Pearls and pitfalls of optical coherence tomography angiography imaging: A review. Ophthalmology and therapy. 2019;**8**:215-226

[40] AAO 2021-2022.12 Retina and Vitreous. Chapter 2 – Diagnostic Approach to Retinal Disease. pp. 21-39

[41] Cennamo G, Carotenuto A, Montorio D, et al. Peripapillary vessel density as early biomarker in multiple sclerosis. Frontiers in Neurology. 2020;**11**:542

Section 4

Era of Artificial Intelligence in Multiple Sclerosis

Chapter 5

Perspective Chapter: Artificial Intelligence in Multiple Sclerosis

Arthi Balasundaram and Mohan Krishna Ghanta

Abstract

In recent times, the words artificial intelligence, machine learning, and deep learning have been making a lot of buzz in different domains and especially in the healthcare sector. In disease areas like multiple sclerosis (MS), these intelligent systems have great potential in aiding the detection and prediction of disease progression and disability, identification of disease subtypes, monitoring, treatment, and novel drug-target identification. The different imaging techniques used to date in multiple sclerosis, various algorithms such as convolutional neural network, Support Vector Machine, long short-term memory networks, JAYA, Random Forest, Naive Bayesian, Sustain, DeepDTnet, and DTINet used in the various domains of multiple sclerosis are explored, along with used cases. Hence it is important for healthcare professionals to have knowledge on artificial intelligence for achieving better healthcare outcomes.

Keywords: AI, disease detection, machine learning, monitoring, MS, treatment

1. Introduction

Artificial intelligence (AI) is progressively being deployed in healthcare, as it becomes more prevalent in recent business and daily activities [1]. AI in healthcare can aid healthcare practitioners with a variety of patient care and administrative operations, helping to strengthen current approaches and overcome difficulties more quickly [2]. Although AI and medical breakthroughs are beneficial to the medical sector, healthcare companies' policies might vary substantially. The most frequent type of AI in healthcare is machine learning (ML). This wide strategy, which is the foundation of several AI and healthcare tools, has several versions. Personalized medicine has been the most widely used application of classical machine learning in the health sector [3]. Supervised learning of AI in healthcare uses machine learning and personalized medicine tools that include data with outcomes for training. The most often used tools of AI in relation to MS disease are ML as well as deep learning (DL) methods [4].

Multiple sclerosis (MS) is a chronic demyelinating autoimmune disorder affecting the central nervous system (CNS) and is prevalent in young adults. Optic neuritis, cerebellar signs, and sensory impairments are common clinical characteristics of MS, especially in recurrent or early phases. Spasticity, ataxia, muscle weakness, and descending tract dysfunctions are all signs of progression [5–7]. With clinical presentation, MS is diagnosed by CNS magnetic resonance imaging (MRI) and cerebrospinal fluid investigation. Earlier studies of AI approaches in distinguishing MS affected

IntechOpen

from healthy subjects or differential diagnoses yielded intriguing results related to diagnostic effectiveness [8]. For the identification of MS lesions in MRI images and the prognosis in MS cases, many AI-based algorithms were suggested [8]. In addition, AI has been used in several trials to anticipate physical as well as cognitive impairment in MS cases [8]. Other data employed in AI tools include Optical coherence tomography, serological, and motor function findings, in addition to MRI findings [9]. The present chapter enables us to understand the role of AI in the detection, prediction, identification of subtypes, monitoring, imaging techniques, drug discovery in MS.

2. Understanding MS using imaging techniques

The development of localized demyelinated lesions known as plaques, which may be detected on standard MRI scans, is the most common characteristic of MS. Now, the focus is mostly on sophisticated MRI techniques that can more reliably disclose the underlying pathology in lesions and seemingly normal CNS structures. The frequently employed imaging techniques for identifying the microscopic progression of pathologies in CNS with high accuracy and precision are Quantitative magnetization transfer imaging (QMTI), proton MRI spectroscopy (MRS), functional MRI (fMRI), diffusion-weighted imaging (DWI), diffusion tensor imaging (DTI), relaxometry, and myelin water fraction (MWF) [10].

Of these, QMTI is considered the advanced technique that detects the association of free protons in edematous fluid with protons linked to myelin membrane constituent molecules. It can also provide information regarding the tissue matrix integrity in MS pathogenesis [11–13]. This technique uses magnetization transfer ratio (MTR) mapping analysis to determine myelin content quantitatively as in normal-appearing white matter changes. Also, magnetization transfer rate (Ksat) and longitudinal relaxation time under MT saturation pulse (T1sat), as well as the computation of T1 longitudinal relaxation time, are used in the QMTI approach to infer neurodegenerative processes. Using QMTI-T1 variables to investigate the degree of lesions in the normal-appearing white matter (NAWM), pathological factors such as neuroinflammation, demyelination, regeneration, gliosis, edema, and axonal degeneration can be monitored more precisely. This method provides for a more accurate evaluation of therapeutic approaches [14–17].

Imaging of the retinal nerve fiber layer (RNFL) and retinal ganglion cells (GCL) has also been suggested for the diagnosis of MS through optical coherence tomography scan (OCT) [18].

3. Role of AI in MS: prediction, detection, and diagnosis of MS

Artificial intelligence (AI) algorithms are a type of machine learning algorithm that has shown great promise in the prediction, detection, and diagnosis of multiple sclerosis (MS). Here are some examples of AI algorithms with potential applications in MS detection, diagnosis, and prediction. The list of algorithms is not limited to the below-mentioned.

3.1 Convolutional neural networks (CNNs)

CNNs are a type of deep learning algorithm used to analyze MRI images and detect MS lesions. These algorithms use a series of convolutional layers to identify features in the images, which are then used to classify the images with or without

MS [19]. The layers of CNN architecture include convolution layers, pooling layers, and fully connected layers. The convolution layer is responsible for the extraction of features from an image. This allows the determination of any abnormalities that are occurring within the image. The pooling layer reduces the dimensionality of the feature maps by down-sampling them, reducing computational complexity before being charted into the final network output [20]. In simpler words, the image becomes smaller, which ultimately reduces the processing time for the subsequent steps executed in the next layer of the neural network [21]. Moreover, recent research interests have involved the development of a novel 14-layer convolutional neural network, for the detection of MS, involving advanced techniques such as dropout, batch normalization, and stochastic pooling. This method has proven to be superior in line with sensitivity, specificity, and accuracy than the traditional AI methods, which are Multiscale AM-FM [22], ARF [23], BWT-logistic regression (LR) [24], 4-level HWT [25], and MBD [26] potentially used for image analysis.

Another novel automated methodology, with higher sensitivity, for the detection of new lesions in images of MS patients has been explored. This algorithm is called 'Fully convolutional neural networks' [FCNNs]. Here, dual streams of FCNNs have been utilized. The initial FCNN network discovers probable candidates, while the second FCNN attempts to detect newer lesions, decreasing the number of false positives. This algorithm helps assess the changes in the lesion volume over two different time points with a faster turnaround time when compared to the manual approach [27]. So, these automated processes are important because they avoid unnecessary exposure to MRI. As per previous studies, it has been emphasized that clinical and radiological results for patients who have not been diagnosed as individuals with MS need to undergo a follow-up MRI of the brain [28]. Overall, in recent times, the convolutional neural network (CNN) has increasingly received attention in image denoising or in other words, deblurring tasks. Image denoising occurs frequently in real-time low-level vision applications. Image denoising continues to be an important subject in the fields of image processing and artificial intelligence because of its ill-posed nature and huge realistic impact [29].

3.2 Support vector machines

Support vector machine (SVM) is a machine learning algorithm that works through regression, classification, and outlier detection of data [30]. The way SVM algorithm in general works is by differentiating two given classes with a hyperplane generation, which divides the classes after the data input, which is transformed mathematically into a high-dimensional space [31]. In a nutshell, this algorithm has been utilized to establish automated disease classifiers [31].

This algorithm has provided high accuracy (98.89%), sensitivity, and positive predictive value for MS diagnosis [32]. There have been instances where plasma levels of nutritional factors such as selenium, vitamin B12, and vitamin D3 as potential markers for MS diagnosis have been explored. Several different algorithm methods were tested as a diagnostic method for nutritional factors based on the MS disease relationship. Out of the several machine learning algorithms, SVM, along with Radial-basis function (RBF) kernel methods, yielded higher accuracy, sensitivity, and predictive values. Basically, these methods work on data analysis and subsequent classification of the same, to determine whether an individual is normal or with MS condition. Some of the other algorithms used in similar aspects are decision tree (DT) and K-nearest neighbor (KNN) [32].

It has been emphasized in existing literature that an early detection or prediction of MS is important for improving the survival of an individual with MS. In lieu of this, many machine learning algorithms have been explored with an expectation to have lesser prediction errors and more accurate classifications of potential MS cases from normal healthy individuals. A few of these algorithms are Naive Bayes (NB), decision trees, random forest (RF), nearest neighbor, AdaBoost, support vector machine (SVM), RBF network, and multilayer perceptron [33].

Another scenario in which the SVM algorithm has been utilized for diagnosing MS is using optical coherence tomography [OCT] data. The retinal structure-based neurodegeneration OCT data parameters used for the analysis are macular thickness and peripapillary region. In fact, analyzing the OCT data for its potential usage as a biomarker in the diagnosis of MS has been an upcoming area in MS research. Usually, MacDonald's Criteria is used for the diagnosis of MS. However, this method may take a longer number of years to arrive at a firm diagnosis from the onset of the disease. In such an instance, it is required to have a more robust and accelerated system that can aid in the early detection of MS, and it is at this juncture that AI-ML-based algorithms play a significant role in executing the same [9].

Another example of the application of an SVM-based technique for diagnosing MS involves MS characterization based on lowered or higher plasma levels of antioxidant or anti-inflammatory biomarkers such as zinc, adiponectin, TRAP, and SH groups and advanced oxidation protein products (AOPP). Here again, the SVM algorithm works by classifying individuals with or without MS based on the higher or lower levels of the above-specified plasma biomarkers data. As a fact, this algorithm has shown higher training and validation accuracy [34].

Application of SVM technique for MS diagnosis based on MRI images has been employed. It has been used to classify based on (a) lesion volume and (b) preprocessed FLAIR (fluid-attenuated inversion recovery) data, which is an advanced form of MRI sequence, perceived to be helpful in the evaluation of MS plaques, lacunar infarction, etc. SVM algorithm, in conjecture with other algorithms such as CNN and layer-wise relevance propagation [LRP], has been used in the diagnosis MS with MRI images. LRP algorithm deals with more understanding and visualizing the intricate inner mechanism of neural networks. To understand LRP better, let us take a hypothetical example where the neural network has predicted a brain lesion from an image of brain tissue. Then, LRP provides a projection of which pixels in the original image had attributed toward the prediction and extent of the same [35]. As a matter of fact, the FLAIR lesion load, which is considered to be one of the significant biomarkers for MS, when combined with the SVM technique, has produced more accurate and robust diagnostic outcomes [36].

3.3 Long short-term memory (LSTM) networks

LSTMs are another type of recurrent neural network-based algorithm, with potential usage in the prediction of the course of MS, based on patient data. This algorithm is trained with clinical data of MS patients and then deployed to newer patient data. In a nutshell, this algorithm analyzes the clinical data of a new patient and provides predictions on whether the patient will progress for example from an initial relapsing-remitting (RR) to the secondary progressive (SP) stage of disease, or not [37]. The variations in clinical data across different time frames, including how they affect prediction outcome, have been employed as feed for classifiers in some research [37–40]. LSTM networks, in particular, enhanced reliability for predictions over extended time periods when used to analyze patient medical history. Since all the data of a patient were combined into a single time series, the amount of data accessible for this strategy was significantly reduced. However, the positive predictive value grew significantly, but at the expense of a decreased sensitivity, or the rate of correctly identifying patients who were becoming worse [37], which would take more time with a human approach, and this tool may help Physicians to save time as well as make decision-making.

3.4 JAYA algorithm

JAYA algorithm is basically used to find the most ideal result for a specific issue. An imaging perspective, this algorithm optimizes MRI parameters, providing better image quality. This algorithm is utilized to spot different tumor types or lesions of varied grades and structures, enabling the treating physician to recognize the tumor or concerned pathological areas and segmentalize more rapidly. Segmentation, in the context of brain MRI, is used for seeing and measuring anatomical aspects of the brain, defining pathological areas, etc. In simpler words, this algorithm is employed for segmenting and extracting abnormal brain portions in brain MRI input data, enabling physicians to arrive at faster and more accurate conclusions and allowing better surgical or treatment planning [41, 42].

So, in the context of MS, the JAYA algorithm and two other techniques, namely MLP and FRFE, have been applied to diagnose MS based on brain MRI images with potentially identifying the MS plaques [43].

3.5 Random forest algorithm

RF is another robust algorithm that provides more accurate predictions [44]. This algorithm, in the context of MS, can be applied for MS diagnosis and disease progression monitoring. Off-late speech patterns have been explored as potential indicators for detecting the presence of neurological disorders [45].

Previous literature has reported that speech discrepancies occur in MS. This feature aids in not only early diagnosis but also in monitoring of MS disease progression. One of the recent research studies involved this concept by making the individual read a text, recording, and storing the same. Then, this algorithm analyzes and provides potential output using the speech recordings derived from MS patients. So here, the algorithm analyzes the speech recordings of healthy and MS patients, which means that the acoustic variables are evaluated statistically, and along with the patient's biometric and health status data, a potential diagnosis and disease progression status of the patient can be derived [45].

3.6 Naive Bayesian networks

Naive Bayesian networks (NBNs) are simple and effective algorithms for disease predictions. It serves like a prediction or probabilistic model for diseases [46]. Bayesian networks are increasingly used as classifiers [47]. So, in MS, Bayesian algorithms analyze a set of clinical and imaging data, which in turn aids in the identification of subtypes. It determines the probability of each patient belonging to a particular MS subtype [47, 48]. Studies suggest that one of the strengths of Bayesian networks is that they can include the gathered knowledge of experts in situations where data are limited and continue to yield significant and accurate decision-support systems [49]. Hence, in this manner, it aids in achieving better clinical outcomes.

3.7 Sustain algorithm

In the field of MS subtype identification, artificial intelligence has a very pivotal role. A newly developed AI algorithm called SUSTAIN has the ability to identify new subtypes of MS. This algorithm basically has the ability to discover data-driven-based subtypes in chronic disorders [48]. In fact SUSTAIN has been utilized in neurodegenerative diseases like Alzheimer's disease, multiple sclerosis, frontotemporal dementia, and progressive lung disease [50].

So, this unsupervised machine learning method groups people with MS into disease subtype categories based on MRI scans, and the algorithm gives a score based on the extent of pathology seen on the MRI scan, subsequently bifurcating the patients into varied categories on certain discrete findings. The uniqueness of SUSTAIN Algorithm is that it can delineate temporal and phenotypic heterogeneity. A set of subtypes is identified by this algorithm, and the subtypes are defined by observing patterns of variations in a group or set of features, for instance, MRI deviations. All of this allows for predicting which MRI-based subtype responds to which particular treatment better, along with taking into account the worsening of Expanded Disability Status Scale (EDSS) as well. So, ultimately, getting the right treatment for the right patient at the right time is achieved [48].

4. Treatment, monitoring, and novel drug-target identification

AI can support decision-making, identify the best course of treatment for a patient, including individualized medications, supervise the collection of clinical data, and use it to ensure subsequent drug development and assist in moving drugs from the research lab to the patients [51, 52]. Various applications of AI in new drug development have been depicted in **Figure 1**. Machine learning (ML) techniques are data-driven methods for creating models of prediction that can recognize patterns and connections in data with relatively little assistance from humans [53, 54]. The use of ML in multiple sclerosis is currently used primarily for categorizing patients into various disease stages [53–55] or for anticipating the transition of disease stage, as

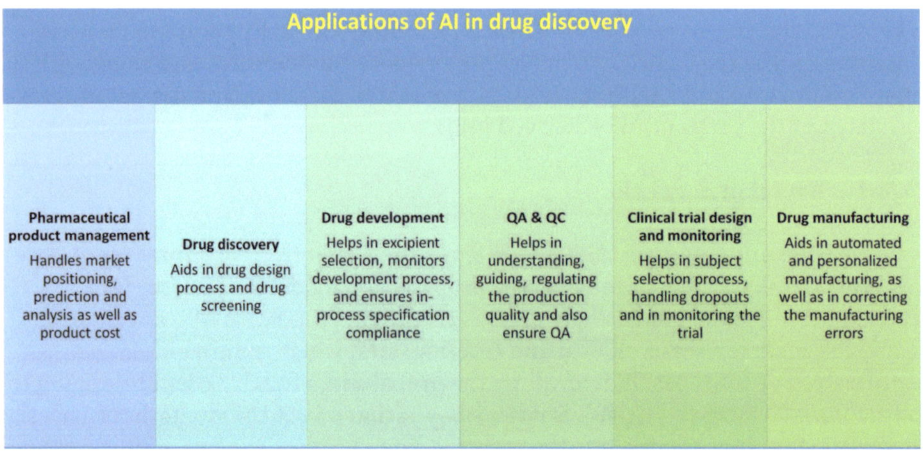

Figure 1.
Scope of AI in drug development process. QA: Quality assurance, QC: Quality control.

well as development of disability [56–58]. It is crucial to identify the illness subtype in new patients. The anticipated time to disease severity progression, especially requiring support for walking, is another important piece of data or parameter to predict [38]. Researchers utilize multidimensional Bayesian network classifiers as they may represent and take advantage of the relationships between both variables, which is important given that we have to forecast two correlated class variables: illness subtype and time to reach a specified severity level. Due to the interpretability of Bayesian networks, the resulting models can also be verified by doctors using their specialized knowledge. A cutting-edge multi-objective method is used to train the classifiers, aiming to simultaneously maximize the accuracy of both class variables [47].

Statistical techniques like linear regression to predict continuous response or LR over binary response anticipation [59], as well as Cox regression or Kaplan–Meier procedures of survival analysis [60], are typically used in predictive models in investigations of prognostic variables that influence the advancement of disabilities. However, these evaluations do not estimate how well they generalize to data that were not utilized for model fitting. In order to predict the Expanded Disability Status Scores (EDSS) at 10 years, for instance, LR was employed to assess brain atrophy as well as lesion burden as prognostic markers. The quality of fit of the model to the data was measured using R2 values, but no prediction of the model's performance using data that were not utilized for model fitting was given [61]. One study used advanced statistical modeling to evaluate the prognostic impact of different clinical measures on disability progression and came to the conclusion that the relatively poor predictive capacity of baseline factors in MS disease progression modeling was confirmed by the inconsistent ranking of prognostic factor importance. One study followed a model that validates data withheld from training in each cycle of 10-CV [62].

Support vector machines may offer a potential way to forecast the path of MS disease and identify individuals who may benefit from intensive treatment approaches by adding short-term clinical as well as brain MRI data, class imbalance correction measures, and misclassification costs [63]. There has been little investigation of machine learning strategies in MS, despite the fact that various research in predicting the course of disease in MS have been done using logistic regression [64], Markov modeling [65–67], and more recently, a Bayesian modeling approach [68]. In order to forecast the progress of the disease in 51 MS patients, one study investigated a neural network computer classifier. Depending on the situation and conditions, an accuracy of >70% may or may not be regarded as a reasonable standard for machine learning [69]. In a different scenario, it was suggested that precise detection of progressive cases without a significant number of false positives is more important so that these patients can receive more aggressive therapies. Therefore, most clinicians may find the predicted accuracy of 81 percent on progressive and 59 percent on nonprogressive using SVM with an expense of 1.5 to be acceptable for clinical purposes. However, it is up to each doctor and patient to decide on this balance [38]. Many investigations mostly centered on quantitative MRI characteristics and clinical data sets. Incorporating biomarker data is unmet. Based on changes in EDSS values over a 5-year period, there may also be variations in the outcome measure for progressive or nonprogressive cases. The weight of progress measured by an increase in EDSS signifies physical disability. The EDSS scale has come under criticism for being fairly insensitive, especially to declines in visual and cognitive abilities. It should be investigated to do further studies using these parameters.

When it comes to patient's disease condition monitoring, one of the words we may often come across is 'wearables. Though short as a word, 'Wearables' are making an immense impact in the world of remote patient monitoring. "Wearables" refers to smallish electronic devices that can be easily put on and off and also be embraced into garments or anybody-based accessories [70].

In MS, the usage of AI-based wearables very much adds onto effective patient monitoring and in turn helps to assess and alter treatment plans for the individual. Gait and cognition are important parameters to be tracked in MS patients and this can be addressed by various intelligent wearables. In fact these wearables can be categorized as software and hardware based. The parameters that can be effectively tracked by these systems are activity levels, fatigue, mood changes, cognitive and mood changes. Adding on as a self-management tool, these systems can aid in timely medication administration and adherence to the same. A few examples of these wearables are 'ActiGraph', 'StepWatch' to monitor activity levels, in terms of the number of steps taken by MS individuals are increasing or decreasing [71]. 'myBETAapp by Bayer', which aims to provide assistance to its autoinjectors BETACONNECT, which helps patients to confidently self-manage their symptoms and dose [72]. 'MyeReport France' is a mobile app for reporting adverse reactions in relapsing remitting MS (RRMS) patients [73]. Another app that aids in monitoring balance and cognition is 'Floodlight' [74].

Another issue that needs to be effectively monitored is the cognitive level of MS patients. As per extensive literature, cognitive impairment is one of the specific features observed in patients with MS, and it is reported that around 45-70% of individuals with MS have cognitive dysfunction [75]. Hence, this can be a potential biomarker for assessing disease status. Recently, a self-administered AI software-based solution, which comprises 5 minutes computerized tests, has been explored to evaluate cognitive dysfunction in MS patients. It uses MLR (multiple linear regression) classifier algorithm to furnish a predictive score in line with the individual's cognitive status [76].

In the new drug discovery process, more than 1060 molecules make up the enormous chemical space, which encourages the creation of many different pharmacological compounds. However, new drug discovery is constrained by a dearth of new technology, rendering it a costly and time-consuming endeavor that may be resolved by applying AI [77]. DeepDTnet is an advanced, network-based DL technology for identifying drug targets as well as drug repurposing that forecasts novel molecular targets within existing pharmaceuticals through systematic embedding of 15 different kinds of chemical, genomic, phenotypic, and cellular networks [78]. DeepDTnet outperforms earlier state-of-the-art network-based as well as conventional machine learning algorithms, according to thorough evaluations, and reveals established drug-target interactions [79]. In one instance, researchers discovered that DTINet performed well when predicting novel targets for medications with high degree in the established drug-target network, but poorly when predicting targets for compounds that had a low degree [80]. DeepDTnet, however, has strong performance in foretelling drug-target interactions across both drugs and targets of high and low degrees. DeepDTnet and DTINet were assessed using a comparable dataset that was previously published in order to accurately compare their performance. DeepDTnet was found to be superior to DTINet as well as NeoDTI, a currently developed successor to DTINet, on both the earlier published dataset and a real-time study data validated drug-target network constructed in a study [81, 82]. Positive-unlabeled matrix completeness as well as autoencoder embedding were two novel deepDTnet components that were used to compare DTINet along with NeoDTI. Both autoencoder embedding along with positive and unlabeled (PU) matrix completeness helped deepDTnet perform better together [78]. This is a systematic deep-learning method that incorporates the biggest biomedical network datasets for target discovery, drug repurposing, and experimental testing of discoveries. By doing this, the translational gap that currently exists between the outcomes of preclinical testing in experimental animals and clinical outcomes in patients can be minimized [80]. The importance of automation will increase as a result of the use of the most recent AI-based technologies, which will additionally reduce the time it takes for new drugs to reach the market while also improving product quality, production process safety, and resource utilization [83]. The biggest concern with implementing these technologies is the potential loss of jobs and the tight rules required for AI implementation. However, these tools are simply meant to facilitate work, not to entirely replace people [84].

5. Conclusions

Artificial intelligence, machine learning, and deep learning in this era are making a significant impact in the healthcare medical vertical. These advanced intelligent systems are being vastly explored in detection, prediction, monitoring, and drug discovery for various disease areas including neurodegenerative and neuroinflammatory conditions such as MS. Though these systems may have noticeable specificity, sensitivity and accuracy in their assessments, further validations and refinements are required to create an extremely robust system. At this juncture, it needs to be emphasized that AI will not replace physicians, but physicians who are not aware of the same may get replaced!

Conflict of interest

"The authors declare no conflict of interest."

Author details

Arthi Balasundaram[1*] and Mohan Krishna Ghanta[2]

1 Neurowyzr Pte Ltd, Singapore

2 Department of Pharmacology, MVJ Medical College and Research Hospital, Karnataka, India

*Address all correspondence to: rtms86@yahoo.com; dr.arthibala@gmail.com

References

[1] Davenport T, Kalakota R. The potential for artificial intelligence in healthcare. Future Healthcare Journal [Internet]. 2019;**6**(2):94-98

[2] Bohr A, Memarzadeh K. The rise of artificial intelligence in healthcare applications. In: Artificial Intelligence in Healthcare. [Internet]. New York, US: Academic Press; 2020. pp. 25-60

[3] Schork NJ. Artificial Intelligence and Personalized Medicine. Cancer Research and Treatment. 2019;**178**:265-283

[4] Sarker IH. Deep learning: A comprehensive overview on techniques, taxonomy, applications and research directions. SN Computer Science. 2021;**2**(6):420

[5] Liu J, Yin L, Dong H, Xu E, Zhang L, Qiao Y, et al. Decreased serum levels of nucleolin protein fragment, as analyzed by bead-based proteomic technology, in multiple sclerosis patients compared to controls. Journal of Neuroimmunology. 2012;**250**(1-2):71-76

[6] Balsundaram A, Chellathai D. Phosphodiesterase 7B1 as therapeutic target for treatment of cognitive dysfunctions in multiple sclerosis. Journal of Pharmacology and Pharmacotherapeutics. 2018;**9**(3):126-130. DOI: 10.4103/jpp.JPP_77_18

[7] Balasundaram A, Chellathai D. Effects of vasicine in neuroinflammatory zebrafish model. Bioinformation. 2023;**19**(5):595-604

[8] Nabizadeh F, Masrouri S, Ramezannezhad E, Ghaderi A, Sharafi AM, Soraneh S, et al. Artificial intelligence in the diagnosis of multiple sclerosis: A systematic review. Multiple Sclerosis and Related Disorders. 2022;**59**:103673

[9] Cavaliere C, Vilades E, Alonso-Rodríguez M, Rodrigo M, Pablo L, Miguel J, et al. Computer-aided diagnosis of multiple sclerosis using a support vector machine and optical coherence tomography features. Sensors. 2019;**19**(23):5323

[10] Fooladi M, Sharini H, Masjoodi S, Khodamoradi E. A novel classification method using effective neural network and quantitative magnetization transfer imaging of brain white matter in relapsing remitting multiple sclerosis. Journal of Biomedical Physics & Engineering. 2018;**8**(4):409-422

[11] Wolff SD, Balaban RS. Magnetization transfer contrast (MTC) and tissue water proton relaxation in vivo. Magnetic Resonance in Medicine. 1989;**10**(1):135-144

[12] Vavasour IM, Laule C, Li DKB, Traboulsee AL, MacKay AL. Is the magnetization transfer ratio a marker for myelin in multiple sclerosis? Journal of Magnetic Resonance Imaging. 2011;**33**(3):713-718

[13] Neema M, Stankiewicz J, Arora A, Guss ZD, Bakshi R. MRI in multiple sclerosis: What's inside the toolbox? Neurotherapeutics. 2007;**4**(4):602-617

[14] Ropele S, Strasser-Fuchs S, Augustin M, Stollberger R, Enzinger C, Hartung HP, et al. A comparison of magnetization transfer ratio, magnetization transfer rate, and the native relaxation time of water protons related to relapsing-remitting multiple sclerosis. AJNR. American Journal of Neuroradiology. 2000;**21**(10):1885-1891

[15] Karampekios S, Papanikolaou N, Papadaki E, Maris T, Uffman K, Spilioti M, et al. Quantification of magnetization transfer rate and native T1 relaxation time of the brain: Correlation with magnetization transfer ratio measurements in patients with multiple sclerosis. Neuroradiology. 2005;**47**(3):189-196

[16] Cercignani M, Symms MR, Schmierer K, Boulby PA, Tozer DJ, Ron M, et al. Three-dimensional quantitative magnetisation transfer imaging of the human brain. NeuroImage. 2005;**27**(2):436-441

[17] Levesque IR, Giacomini PS, Narayanan S, Ribeiro LT, Sled JG, Arnold DL, et al. Quantitative magnetization transfer and myelin water imaging of the evolution of acute multiple sclerosis lesions. Magnetic Resonance in Medicine. 2010;**63**(3):633-640

[18] Garcia-Martin E, Pablo LE, Herrero R, Ara JR, Martin J, Larrosa JM, et al. Neural networks to identify multiple sclerosis with optical coherence tomography. Acta Ophthalmologica. 2013;**91**(8): e628-e634

[19] Yamashita R, Nishio M, Do RKG, Togashi K. Convolutional neural networks: An overview and application in radiology. Insights into Imaging [Internet]. 2018;**9**(4):611-629

[20] Rguibi Z, Hajami A, Zitouni D, Elqaraoui A, Bedraoui A. CXAI: Explaining convolutional neural networks for medical imaging diagnostic. Electronics (Basel). 2022;**11**(11):1775

[21] Alzubaidi L, Zhang J, Humaidi AJ, Al-Dujaili A, Duan Y, Al-Shamma O, et al. Review of deep learning: Concepts, CNN architectures, challenges, applications, future directions. Journal of Big Data. 2021;**8**(1):53

[22] Murray V, Rodriguez P, Pattichis MS. Multiscale AM-FM demodulation and image reconstruction methods with improved accuracy. IEEE Transactions on Image Processing. 2010;**19**(5):1138-1152

[23] Nayak DR, Dash R, Majhi B. Brain MR image classification using two-dimensional discrete wavelet transform and AdaBoost with random forests. Neurocomputing. 2016;**177**:188-197

[24] Wang SH, Zhan TM, Chen Y, Zhang Y, Yang M, Lu HM, et al. Multiple sclerosis detection based on biorthogonal wavelet transform, RBF kernel principal component analysis, and logistic regression. IEEE Access. 2016;**4**:7567-7576

[25] Wu X, Lopez M. Multiple sclerosis slice identification by Haar wavelet transform and logistic regression. In: Proceedings of the Advances in Materials, Machinery, Electrical Engineering (AMMEE 2017). Paris, France: Atlantis Press; 2017. pp. 50-55

[26] Zhang YD, Zhang Y, Phillips P, Dong Z, Wang S. Synthetic minority oversampling technique and fractal dimension for identifying multiple sclerosis. Fractals. 2017;**25**(04):1740010

[27] Salem M, Ryan MA, Oliver A, Hussain KF, Lladó X. Improving the detection of new lesions in multiple sclerosis with a cascaded 3D fully convolutional neural network approach. Frontiers in Neuroscience. 2022;**16**:1007619

[28] Rovira À, Wattjes MP, Tintoré M, Tur C, Yousry TA, Sormani MP, et al. MAGNIMS consensus guidelines on the use of MRI in multiple sclerosis—Clinical implementation in the diagnostic

process. Nature Reviews. Neurology. 2015;**11**(8):471-482

[29] Ilesanmi AE, Ilesanmi TO. Methods for image denoising using convolutional neural network: A review. Complex & Intelligent Systems. 2021;**7**(5):2179-2198

[30] Mourão-Miranda J, Hardoon DR, Hahn T, Marquand AF, Williams SCR, Shawe-Taylor J, et al. Patient classification as an outlier detection problem: An application of the one-class support vector machine. NeuroImage. 2011;**58**(3):793-804

[31] Yu W, Liu T, Valdez R, Gwinn M, Khoury MJ. Application of support vector machine modeling for prediction of common diseases: The case of diabetes and pre-diabetes. BMC Medical Informatics and Decision Making. 2010;**10**(1):16

[32] Sharifmousavi SS, Borhani MS. Support vectors machine-based model for diagnosis of multiple sclerosis using the plasma levels of selenium, vitamin B12, and vitamin D3. Informatics in Medicine Unlocked. 2020;**20**:100382

[33] Seccia R, Romano S, Salvetti M, Crisanti A, Palagi L, Grassi F. Machine learning use for prognostic purposes in multiple sclerosis. Life. 2021;**11**(2):122

[34] Mezzaroba L, Simão ANC, Oliveira SR, Flauzino T, Alfieri DF, de Carvalho Jennings Pereira WL, et al. Antioxidant and anti-inflammatory diagnostic biomarkers in multiple sclerosis: A machine learning study. Molecular Neurobiology. 2020;**57**(5):2167-2178

[35] Zang B, Ding L, Feng Z, Zhu M, Lei T, Xing M, et al. CNN-LRP: Understanding convolutional neural networks performance for target recognition in SAR images. Sensors. 2021;**21**(13):4536

[36] Eitel F, Soehler E, Bellmann-Strobl J, Brandt AU, Ruprecht K, Giess RM, et al. Uncovering convolutional neural network decisions for diagnosing multiple sclerosis on conventional MRI using layer-wise relevance propagation. NeuroImage: Clinical. 2019;**24**:102003

[37] Seccia R, Gammelli D, Dominici F, Romano S, Landi AC, Salvetti M, et al. Considering patient clinical history impacts performance of machine learning models in predicting course of multiple sclerosis. PLoS One. 2020;**15**(3):e0230219

[38] Zhao Y, Healy BC, Rotstein D, Guttmann CRG, Bakshi R, Weiner HL, et al. Exploration of machine learning techniques in predicting multiple sclerosis disease course. PLoS One. 2017;**12**:e0174866. DOI: 10.1371/journal.pone.0174866

[39] Zhao Y, Investigators S, Wang T, Bove R, Cree B, Henry R, et al. Ensemble learning predicts multiple sclerosis disease course in the SUMMIT study. NPJ Digital Medicine. 2020;**3**:135. DOI: 10.1038/s41746-020-00338-8

[40] Pinto MF, Oliveira H, Batista S, Cruz L, Pinto M, Correia I, et al. Prediction of disease progression and outcomes in multiple sclerosis with machine learning. Scientific Reports. 2020;**10**:21038. DOI: 10.1038/s41598-020-78212-6

[41] Despotović I, Goossens B, Philips W. MRI segmentation of the human brain: Challenges, methods, and applications. Computational and Mathematical Methods in Medicine. 2015;**2015**:1-23

[42] Kaur K, Kaur Walia G, Kaur J. Neural network ensemble and Jaya algorithm

based diagnosis of brain tumor using MRI images. Journal of The Institution of Engineers (India): Series B. 2018;**99**(5):509-517

[43] Wang SH, Cheng H, Phillips P, Zhang YD. Multiple sclerosis identification based on fractional Fourier entropy and a modified Jaya algorithm. Entropy. 2018;**20**(4):254

[44] Omar KS, Islam MN, Khan NS. Exploring tree-based machine learning methods to predict autism spectrum disorder. In: Neural Engineering Techniques for Autism Spectrum Disorder. New York, US: Academic Press; 2021. pp. 165-183

[45] Svoboda E, Bořil T, Rusz J, Tykalová T, Horáková D, Guttmann CRG, et al. Assessing clinical utility of machine learning and artificial intelligence approaches to analyze speech recordings in multiple sclerosis: A pilot study. Computers in Biology and Medicine. 2022;**148**:105853

[46] Langarizadeh M, Moghbeli F. Applying Naive Bayesian networks to disease prediction: A systematic review. Acta Informatica Medica. 2016;**24**(5):364

[47] Rodriguez JD, Perez A, Arteta D, Tejedor D, Lozano JA. Using multidimensional Bayesian network classifiers to assist the treatment of multiple sclerosis. IEEE Transactions on Systems, Man, and Cybernetics, Part C (Applications and Reviews). 2012;**42**(6):1705-1715

[48] Eshaghi A, Young AL, Wijeratne PA, Prados F, Arnold DL, Narayanan S, et al. Identifying multiple sclerosis subtypes using unsupervised machine learning and MRI data. Nature Communications. 2021;**12**(1):2078

[49] McLachlan S, Dube K, Hitman GA, Fenton NE, Kyrimi E. Bayesian networks in healthcare: Distribution by medical condition. Artificial Intelligence in Medicine. 2020;**107**:101912. DOI: 10.1016/j.artmed.2020.101912. Epub 2020 Jun 10

[50] Aksman LM, Wijeratne PA, Oxtoby NP, Eshaghi A, Shand C, Altmann A, et al. pySuStaIn: A python implementation of the subtype and stage inference algorithm. SoftwareX. 2021;**16**:100811

[51] Duch W, Swaminathan K, Meller J. Artificial intelligence approaches for rational drug design and discovery. Current Pharmaceutical Design. 2007;**13**(14):1497-1508

[52] Blasiak A, Khong J, Kee T, Curate AI. Optimizing personalized medicine with artificial intelligence. SLAS Technology: Translating Life Sciences Innovation. 2020;**25**(2):95-105

[53] Zhong J, Chen DQ, Nantes JC, Holmes SA, Hodaie M, Koski L. Combined structural and functional patterns discriminating upper limb motor disability in multiple sclerosis using multivariate approaches. Brain Imaging and Behavior. 2017;**11**(3):754-768

[54] Zurita M, Montalba C, Labbé T, Cruz JP, Dalboni da Rocha J, Tejos C, et al. Characterization of relapsing-remitting multiple sclerosis patients using support vector machine classifications of functional and diffusion MRI data. NeuroImage. Clinical. 2018;**20**:724-730

[55] Ion-Mărgineanu A, Kocevar G, Stamile C, Sima DM, Durand-Dubief F, Van Huffel S, et al. Machine learning approach for classifying multiple sclerosis courses by combining clinical data with lesion loads and magnetic resonance metabolic features. Frontiers in Neuroscience. 2017;**11**:398

[56] Wottschel V, Alexander DC, Kwok PP, Chard DT, Stromillo ML, De Stefano N, et al. Predicting outcome in clinically isolated syndrome using machine learning. NeuroImage. Clinical. 2015;**7**:281-287

[57] Bendfeldt K, Taschler B, Gaetano L, Madoerin P, Kuster P, Mueller-Lenke N, et al. MRI-based prediction of conversion from clinically isolated syndrome to clinically definite multiple sclerosis using SVM and lesion geometry. Brain Imaging and Behavior. 2019;**13**(5):1361-1374

[58] Zhang H, Alberts E, Pongratz V, Mühlau M, Zimmer C, Wiestler B, et al. Predicting conversion from clinically isolated syndrome to multiple sclerosis–An imaging-based machine learning approach. NeuroImage. Clinical. 2019;**21**:101593

[59] Tripepi G, Jager KJ, Dekker FW, Zoccali C. Linear and logistic regression analysis. Kidney International. 2008;**73**(7):806-810

[60] Bewick V, Cheek L, Ball J. Statistics review 12: Survival analysis. Critical Care. 2004;**8**(5):389

[61] Popescu V, Agosta F, Hulst HE, Sluimer IC, Knol DL, Sormani MP, et al. Brain atrophy and lesion load predict long term disability in multiple sclerosis. Journal of Neurology, Neurosurgery, and Psychiatry. 2013;**84**(10):1082-1091

[62] Law MT, Traboulsee AL, Li DK, Carruthers RL, Freedman MS, Kolind SH, et al. Machine learning in secondary progressive multiple sclerosis: An improved predictive model for short-term disability progression. Multiple Sclerosis Journal - Experimental, Translational and Clinical. 2019;**5**(4):205521731988598

[63] Wolpert DH. The lack of a priori distinctions between learning algorithms. Neural Computation. 1996;**8**(7):1341-1390

[64] Bosma LV, Kragt JJ, Knol DL, Polman CH, Uitdehaag BM. Clinical scales in progressive MS: Predicting long-term disability. Multiple Sclerosis Journal. 2012;**18**(3):345-350

[65] Gauthier SA, Mandel M, Guttmann CRG, Glanz BI, Khoury SJ, Betensky RA, et al. Predicting short-term disability in multiple sclerosis. Neurology. 2007;**68**(24):2059-2065

[66] Wolfson C, Confavreux C. Improvements to a simple Markov model of the natural history of multiple sclerosis. Neuroepidemiology. 1987;**6**(3):101-115

[67] Wolfson C, Confavreux C. A Markov model of the natural history of multiple sclerosis. Neuroepidemiology. 1985;**4**(4):227-239

[68] Bergamaschi R, Quaglini S, Trojano M, Amato MP, Tavazzi E, Paolicelli D, et al. Early prediction of the long term evolution of multiple sclerosis: The Bayesian risk estimate for multiple sclerosis (BREMS) score. Journal of Neurology, Neurosurgery, and Psychiatry. 2006;**78**(7):757-759

[69] Bejarano B, Bianco M, Gonzalez-Moron D, Sepulcre J, Goñi J, Arcocha J, et al. Computational classifiers for predicting the short-term course of multiple sclerosis. BMC Neurology. 2011;**11**(1):67

[70] Smuck M, Odonkor CA, Wilt JK, Schmidt N, Swiernik MA. The emerging clinical role of wearables: Factors for successful implementation in healthcare. NPJ Digital Medicine. 2021;**4**(1):45

[71] Sandroff BM, Motl RW, Pilutti LA, Learmonth YC, Ensari I, Dlugonski D,

et al. Accuracy of StepWatchTM and ActiGraph accelerometers for measuring steps taken among persons with multiple sclerosis. PLoS One. 2014;**9**(4):e93511

[72] Alexander S, Peryer G, Gray E, Barkhof F, Chataway J. Wearable technologies to measure clinical outcomes in multiple sclerosis: A scoping review. Multiple Sclerosis Journal. 2021;**27**(11):1643-1656

[73] Defer G, Le Caignec F, Fedrizzi S, Montastruc F, Chevanne D, Parienti JJ, et al. Dedicated mobile application for drug adverse reaction reporting by patients with relapsing remitting multiple sclerosis (Vigip-SEP study): Study protocol for a randomized controlled trial. Trials. 2018;**19**(1):174

[74] Montalban X, Graves J, Midaglia L, Mulero P, Julian L, Baker M, et al. A smartphone sensor-based digital outcome assessment of multiple sclerosis. Multiple Sclerosis Journal. 2022;**28**(4):654-664

[75] Elshebawy H, Fahmy EM, Elfayoumy NM, Abdelalim AM, Ismail RS. Clinical predictors to cognitive impairment in multiple sclerosis patients. The Egyptian Journal of Neurology, Psychiatry and Neurosurgery. 2021;**57**(1):38

[76] Khaligh-Razavi SM, Sadeghi M, Khanbagi M, Kalafatis C, Nabavi SM. A self-administered, artificial intelligence (AI) platform for cognitive assessment in multiple sclerosis (MS). BMC Neurology. 2020;**20**(1):193

[77] Mak KK, Pichika MR. Artificial intelligence in drug development: Present status and future prospects. Drug Discovery Today. 2019;**24**(3):773-780

[78] Simm J, Klambauer G, Arany A, Steijaert M, Wegner JK, Gustin E, et al. Repurposing high-throughput image assays enables biological activity prediction for drug discovery. Cell Chemical Biology. 2018;**25**(5):611-618.e3

[79] Xia Z, Wu LY, Zhou X, Wong ST. Semi-supervised drug-protein interaction prediction from heterogeneous biological spaces. BMC Systems Biology. 2010;**4**(S2):S6

[80] Zeng X, Zhu S, Lu W, Liu Z, Huang J, Zhou Y, et al. Target identification among known drugs by deep learning from heterogeneous networks. Chemical Science. 2020;**11**(7):1775-1797

[81] Wan F, Hong L, Xiao A, Jiang T, Zeng J. NeoDTI: Neural integration of neighbor information from a heterogeneous network for discovering new drug-target interactions. Bioinformatics. 2019;**35**(1):104-111

[82] Cheng F. In silico oncology drug repositioning and polypharmacology. Methods in Molecular Biology. 2019;**1878**:243-261

[83] Jämsä-Jounela SL. Future trends in process automation. Annual Reviews in Control. 2007;**31**(2):211-220

[84] Dwivedi YK, Hughes L, Ismagilova E, Aarts G, Coombs C, Crick T, et al. Artificial intelligence (AI): Multidisciplinary perspectives on emerging challenges, opportunities, and agenda for research, practice and policy. International Journal of Information Management. 2021;**57**:101994

Section 5

Neurocognition and Neuroimmunology in Multiple Sclerosis

Chapter 6

Cognitive Impairments in Early Multiple Sclerosis

Raphiq Ibrahim

Abstract

Over the past few decades clinical and research awareness has grown about the nature and prevalence of cognitive disorders in multiple sclerosis (MS). It is assumed that 65% of hospitalized MS patients develop cognitive impairments which have consistently demonstrated a pattern of decline in the following areas: attention working memory executive functions and verbal episodic memory. This chapter reviews the evidence for its associated comorbidities which may address early in the disease course that supports the importance for early recognition and management of cognitive impairment in MS before it becomes an irreversible entity. The focus is on three areas of inquiry: The first aims to provide a description of cognitive impairment in MS at all disease stages and in all subtypes. The second tried to evaluate the clinical imaging and neuroanatomical aspects. And the third focuses on cognitive assessment therapy and rehabilitation based on the literature.

Keywords: multiple sclerosis, cognitive impairment, comorbidities, assessment, imaging, memory disorder, therapy, rehabilitation

1. Introduction

Deficits of diseases of the brain have been extensively characterized in the last decades. However, few studies have examined their associated cognitive impairments. In the last decade, interest has focused on the cognitive impairments that develop following encephalitis (see, [1]) and multiple sclerosis (MS) [2, 3]. The symptoms of MS disease impairments were determined mainly by examining the hospital records of those previously admitted with degree of central nervous system damage (cerebral inflammation), who were assessed after detecting motor, and other neurological dysfunction. We now know that cognitive impairment associated with multiple sclerosis can have many faces, and like other symptoms of multiple sclerosis, the cognitive deficits are highly variable. Although cognitive impairment in MS impacts negatively on many patients at all disease stages and in all subtypes, full clinical cognitive assessment is expensive, requiring time and expert staff. In addition, standardized tests are not available for all languages and cultures. This chapter deals with these stages and subtypes, clinical assessment, imaging and neuroanatomical aspects, therapy, and rehabilitation based on the literature and subjective clinical experience and follow-up.

2. Background

Multiple sclerosis (MS) is a chronic disease affecting the central nervous system (including the brain, optic nerves, and spinal cord). It is characterized by the destruction of the insulating myelin layer of nerve fibers within the brain. The classical course of the disease evolves when the immune system attacks the nerve cells. Usually, the initial stage of the disease alternates between inflammatory autoimmune attacks on myelin by infiltrating T-cells and periods of remission and partial recovery, called relapsing-remitting MS (RRMS) [4]. Two major courses of multiple sclerosis have been described: an offensive course and the preliminary chronic course. The myelin sheath surrounds the nerve cells and serves the dual purpose of augmenting the conduction of nervous signals. Once the myelin sheath is damaged, nerve signaling is impaired, and this malfunction leads to various symptoms such as numbness, fatigue, weakness, blurry vision, and cognitive dysfunctions (high-level functions that include: information processing speed, attention, memory, and executive function). There is a broad-spectrum symptom, whose manifestation depends on the degree of brain damage and the neuroanatomical scattering. According to Lublin et al. [5], the frequency of relapses can vary from patient to patient. While most cases of RRMS are mild and the symptoms could last for a long time, it can be followed by a progressive stage of irreversible degeneration of demyelinated and exposed nerve cells, called secondary progressive MS (SPMS). In some cases, the disease is progressive from the onset. This type of MS is called primary progressive MS (PPMS). These destructive processes cause severe symptoms including blurred vision, loss of balance, poor coordination, slurred speech, tremors, numbness, fatigue, paralysis, and dysfunctions in memory and concentration. This chapter explores the way that MS affects high-level functions with a focus on memory and executive functions according to the stages and subtypes of multiple sclerosis.

3. Cognitive impairment in multiple sclerosis

Over the past few decades, clinical and research interest has grown about the nature and prevalence of cognitive impairment associated with multiple sclerosis. Cognitive impairment has been reported in all stages and subtypes of multiple sclerosis. The severity and type of cognitive impairment vary between individuals and can be observed in both early and progressive stages. The cognitive impairment, which is based on the findings of many studies, has consistently demonstrated a pattern of decline in the following areas: ability to maintain attention over time, retrieving information received after time delay, information processing speed, spatial visual perception, abstraction ability, and verbal fluency.

Prevalence studies of community and clinical samples indicate that 53–65% of hospitalized MS patients develop cognitive impairments [6]. Cognitive impairment contributes significantly to the patients' disability status, but there is no significant correlation between cognitive impairment and physical disability [7]. However, it is known that cognitive impairment increases morbidity in patients and is associated with a decrease in participation and functioning of daily life activities, such as driving, making medical decisions, adhering to treatment, and managing finances and work. Furthermore, cognitive impairment appears to be associated with increased unemployment rates and lower quality of life. For example, 7 years after diagnosis, only 54.4% of the MS population remains employed. This is associated with the presence of cognitive impairment (CI) at the time of, or shortly after, MS diagnosis [8]. The most common cognitive deficits in MS are slowed cognitive processing speed and episodic memory decline in addition to difficulties in executive function, verbal fluency, and visuospatial analysis. Cognitive decline often emerges early in disease, but impairment is more prevalent and may differ qualitatively (e.g., working memory deficits) among patients in progressive stage.

In view of the fact that memory disorder is one of the most common symptoms reported in MS patients, it is obvious that this chapter focuses on this and related function according to stages and subtypes of multiple sclerosis. As the nature and source of memory impairment are still in debate in the professional literature, the main question in this regard is whether memory loss is caused as a result of a deficit in acquisition process, encoding deficit, or retrieval ability. In a number of studies, it has been found that while MS patients demonstrate relatively normal short-term memory functions, they show difficulties in remembering long-term information, and the difficulties increase as they are more exposed to various distractions (interference) [9, 10]. In the field of verbal memory, difficulties in spontaneous retrieval are described with an improvement in the performance of recognition tasks. In examining nonverbal memory tasks, shortages in the recall of visual information were demonstrated. It has been found that when MS patients are compared to control subjects, they show poorer performance in remembering practical forms and in remembering their spatial location [9]. Ron et al [10] even argued that memory impairments in MS patients are more prominent in the visual stimuli than in the verbal stimuli. In the same study, a correlation was found between cognitive decline and the extent of brain damage and the duration of the disease. Regarding the effect of different disease characteristics on memory functions, [11] found that MS patients in a progressive stage show deficiency in information acquisition. However, their performance was not found significantly different in the identification tasks than those of the control subjects. Most of the studies conducted among the MS patient population were built on the awareness level paradigm when acquiring new information. A later study conducted by [12] examined memory functions under different conditions: explicit vs implicit memory. In their study, they used the task of completing the roots of the word, in order to separate explicit and implicit learning. It was found that while MS subjects diagnosed as having cognitive decline, they showed normal performance in tasks that tested for non-intentional learning and poor performance in tasks that test intentional learning. MS patients not diagnosed as suffering from cognitive decline performed all tasks at a level similar to that of a group of control subjects. This study reinforces the assumption of [13] that an *emplicit* process of acquiring information is based on conserved cortical structures, with a deliberate learning process more closely linked to the subcortical structures. Namely, the main cause of implicit learning disorder in MS patients suffering from cognitive decline is due to a disconnection between the cortical regions and subcortical structures. In regard to performance in autobiographical memory in multiple sclerosis [14], found that close to 66% of MS patients exhibit autobiographical memory impairments, with the ability to remember episodic autobiographical events being more impaired than the ability to remember semantic autobiographical information. It should be noted that this study examined patients at an advanced stage of the disease a factor that may explain the severity of the deficiencies that were demonstrated. A supporting result came from clinical studies with head injury patients. De Sonneville et al. [15] used a neuropsychological battery designed to test for split attention, ability to focus attention, ability to maintain an attention over time, and executive functions. Significant deficiencies were found in MS patients compared to control group in all areas examined. In addition, patients in the progressive disease stage were significantly inferior to the group of patients with relapsing-remitting disease stage. Along with the previous results demonstrated by [16], a significant correlation was found between the subtype and duration of the disease and the decline in cognitive functions. The Paced Auditory Serial Addition Test (PASAT) task is the most used task in trying to detect defects in the areas of working memory and information processing, and it has been included as a central part for these purposes in a specific battery designed for MS patients (MSFC). Fisk and Archibald [17] pointed out a certain difficulty in interpreting the results of this test because an increase in the level of complexity of the task leads to an executive strategy of chunking, which may disguise the true ability. Reporting bugs in areas that test visual information processing, Laatu et al. [18] used visually displayed objects in order to detect whether there is a deficiency in specific information processing stages that may be present in MS patients. The results revealed that MS patients with a diagnosed cognitive decline had difficulty with tasks that required the distinction and identification of visual forms (early stage of information processing) and the ability to associate objects according to semantic-lexical information. Due to the great variability between different patient groups, it has been hypothesized that even cognitively normal MS patients may have difficulty in processing visual information.

It is important to note that standard neuropsychological tests in some cases fail to detect clinically emergent cognitive deficits and cognitive complaints reported by patients, which can be confounded by other subjective symptoms (comorbidities) (see, [7]). That is, cognitive functions can be affected by emotional stress, depression, sleep disorders, menopause, aging, or fatigue. Furthermore, some prescription treatment drugs can impair cognitive performance. But this issue falls out the scope of this work.

3.1 Cognitive assessment

Although a high incidence of CI is recognized in advanced stages of MS, the point at which CI first appears is not clearly defined. It is likely that the disease is not diagnosed in the early stages even after neuropsychological assessment, and indeed the presence of CI does not seem to be highly correlated with the its duration.

However, accurate measurement is an important aspect of comprehensive patient management. Routine clinical evaluation by the neurologist lacks sensitivity in detecting CI, compared to standard neuropsychological tests. This is due to both patient underreporting and the use of brief cognitive assessment measures in clinical practice. The most commonly used are the Mini-Mental State Examination (MMSE) and the Montreal Cognitive Assessments, which test mainly for cortical functions; short-term memory loss, aphasia, apraxia, construction, and orientation, areas that are usually affected in dementia, but not in MS. With only limited testing of attention and executive functions, they are not sensitive or specific tests for CI in MS.

There is no single test that measures cognitive problems in MS. Some screening tools are available, but none of them are perfect. Research studies often use the PASAT (Paced Auditory Serial Addition Test). It takes a few minutes and consists of a task that measures addition and repetition of previous numbers. It may be moderately stressful. A formal neuropsychological examination is the best test for assessing disturbing cognitive changes in MS. During a neuropsychological evaluation, multiple tests are used to measure memory, attention, and many other parts of cognition. The speed of cognitive processing is usually estimated as the amount of work done within a time limit (e.g., the number of items completed). There are number of cognitive batteries developed for MS, include tests of processing episodic memory (e.g., the amount of information learned and remembered: words, visual stimuli), speed, memory, and other functions managed separately by skilled professionals. We critically reviewed the most common tasks and identified the Symbol Literature Test (SDMT), the Short Vision-Spatial Memory Test (BVMT-R), and the Selective Reminder Test or Verbal Learning Test in California-II (CVLT-II) as the tasks that are most sensitive and the most available today for cognitive monitoring in multiple sclerosis. SDMT is the most sensitive, probably because good performance depends on a number of functions affected by MS (mainly processing speed, but also memory and visual scanning).

Although MS is short on neuropsychological standards, the need for even 15 minutes of one-on-one testing for each patient is impractical, so cognitive monitoring is not part of standard MS treatment. A computerized test may be a worthy alternative to a conventional paper and pencil evaluation. For example, the Processing Speed Test (PST) is a tablet-based test designed according to the SDMT (and part of MS Performance). The quality of the battery used for assessment in MS should be determined based on the following: standardization, ability to differentiate the MS population from controls, test-retest reliability, availability of normative data, and learning effects.

The Brief Neuropsychological Test of Repetition Battery (BRB-N) consists of five different neuropsychological tests: selective recall, spatial recall, symbolic digit modes, rhythmic serial auditory addition, and word list generation tests. It has been validated as a sensitive measure of early CI in MS, with a sensitivity of 71% and a specificity of 94%, in distinguishing cognitively impaired from cognitively intact MS patients. It takes 45 minutes to administer and requires staff trained in neuropsychology. PASAT is particularly subject to learning effects when repeated, which usually do not stabilize until repeated at least three times in a participant. Both are the most commonly used and validated neuropsychological batteries for MS. They are comparable in their discriminative power, with equal abilities to discriminate between MS patients and healthy controls. Because both are time-consuming and require specialized materials and experienced neuropsychologists to administer and interpret, they are not used in routine clinical practice.

A diagnosis of probable mild-to-moderate cognitive impairment may trigger a person with MS to engage in a more "brain-healthy" lifestyle, if they have not already done so [7]. Marrie and Horwitz [7] claimed that although the interaction between comorbidities and chronic diseases is strong, the effect of comorbidities receives little attention in many chronic diseases. Patterns of cognitive impairment in multiple sclerosis and clinical assessment are present in all subtypes of MS, but are more common and more severe in progressive rather than relapsing MS.

To summerize, MS can induce different types of damage to the cognitive system. Although the ability to detect cognitive difficulties has improved over the past few years, there are many patients who are not diagnosed. Morever, in patients with multiple sclerosis and cognitive impairment, the full etiology remains unclear, as little is still known about their relative contribution to the underlying process of cognitive impairment. There is also a poor correlation between symptoms of cognitive impairment and conventional MRI measures of structural damage. At present, neurologists perform short assessments as a screening tool for cognitive impairment in MS. This is because a formal cognitive assessment done by neuropsychologists may be expensive and require several hours, expert staff, and special equipment. Furthermore, the neuropsychological assessment should take into account comorbidity and distinguish between cognitive impairment and other causes of perceived impairment, including anxiety, depression, and quality of life. Neuropsychological batteries yield quantitative values, and impairment is generally defined as performance below the selected threshold (e.g., 1.5 SD below norm). However, the definitions of impairment have changed between studies, affecting the prevalence of impairment. Future work should better characterize groups as those with isolated or combined deficits (phenotypes, e.g., impaired memory but intact speed; impaired speed and memory) and use purer indices of each cognitive domain (e.g., latent variables or complex domain scores).

3.2 Imaging and neuroanatomical aspects of CI in MS

Recent developments in magnetic resonance imaging (MRI) techniques show a better association with CI than conventional measures of demyelination and offer insights into its pathogenesis. The literature suggests patterns of CI in MS associated to radiological findings. The focus is particularly on the evidence in the early stages of MS after diagnosis.

In fact, there is an increasing arsenal of function-based MRI assessment protocols (e.g., functional and effective connectivities (EC) and the generation of dysconnectivity maps) providing insight into the causal relations that may be impaired [19]. Effective connectivity (EC) estimations as derived from fMRI allow quantification of information flows in neural networks. Hence, EC is able to explore causal effects between cortical areas, which are highly relevant for biological network behavior and can be traced longitudinally to depict brain reorganization processes in brain diseases [20, 21].

The first evidence for the existence of cerebral compensatory processes in multiple sclerosis was received about four decades ago. In 1984, Mintun, Raichle, Martin, and Herscovitch examined a patient with a right demyelinating focus documented on a CT scan. This focus was demonstrated as a hypometabolic region on PET examination and was accompanied by a hypermetabolic region in the left hemisphere. There are neuroanatomical correlations of existing cognitive impairments (e.g., thalamus), but it is unclear whether such correlations are directly underlying the impairments or are reliable proxies for total (or other) brain damage, mediating links to cognition [22]. According to Ross and Ebner [22], the thalamus is very sensitive to retrograde degeneration and has a better scan-to-scan reliability than other structures. The thalamus volume constitutes a good measure of disease load across patients with variable central nervous system damage even it does not directly underlie a specific deficit (e.g., memory). In that regard, a large prospective longitudinal study with multimodal neural imaging needed to carefully document temporary correlations of specific cognitive impairments that arise with changes in specific brain structures and functions, thus informing advanced models of disease-related impairments that will help identify therapeutic goals. Other researchers have suggested that longitudinal work may help establish transverse associations between memory impairments and changes in the hippocampus [23]. There is also a growing body of literature of neurostimulation employed for memory improvement to enhance lateralization and functional connectivity [24]. Veréb and his colleagues [24] confirm previous descriptions of Resting State Networks[1] (RSN) dysfunction in relapsing-remitting MS and show that altered functional connectivity lateralization patterns of RSNs might contribute to cognitive performance and structural demodulation even in patients with mild clinical symptoms.

[1] Resting-State Setworks (RSNs) refer to distant brain regions display synchronous BOLD signal oscillations, testifying to functional connectivity between regions and forming intrinsic functional networks. RSNs are related to cognition and their alteration has been linked to various brain pathologies.

Huber et al. [25] examined a group of MS patients using neuropsychological tests and MRI. They found that only 28% of patients met the criteria for dementia, but the number and location of cortical lesions were no different from dementia patients compared to 72% of non-dementia patients. A further study by Steffan [26] using fMRI found differences in activation patterns when performing an attention task in MS patients compared to controls. In control subjects, an activation focus was found in the right frontal area, whereas in MS patients, the activation was more diffuse and was observed in both the right and left frontal areas. This finding is interpreted as an expression of a compensatory process that plays an important role already in the early stages of the disease (Mintun, Raichle, Martin & Herscovitch, 1984). In a similar technique used by Zivadinov and his colleagues [27], they found an indication of metabolic imbalance in brain tissue, even in disease stages that had no clinical manifestation (without permanent neurological damage). Furthermore, a correlation was demonstrated between the degree of brain parenchyma damage and cognitive impairments, demonstrating important aspects that may contribute to both understanding the disease itself and the nature of its effects on cognitive processes. In general, even today we are still talking about the following factors and their important role in the pathogenesis of cognitive decline in MS: several brain lesions, intensity of pathological damage to brain tissue around lesions (parenchime), and axonal loss. Both clinical and associated radiological findings will apply particularly to processes involved in the early stages of MS after diagnosis.

4. Cognitive therapy and rehabilitation

Neuropsychological rehabilitation is currently the mainstay of treatment for cognitive disorders in multiple sclerosis. Training that improves cognitive function can significantly improve the quality of life of a person with multiple sclerosis. There is also a chance to support prevention of cognitive decline through, among other things, interventions and healthy lifestyles that promote brain maintenance. In cases of relapsing-remitting attacks, drug treatments for multiple sclerosis may help stabilize and possibly improve cognition if the disease is caught early enough.

The literature shows that rehabilitative cognitive therapy may be beneficial to the overall picture and make it easier to deal with difficulties in daily life. However, there are few controlled studies on the effectiveness of MS treatment, and these studies have provided limited evidence that disease-modifying therapies are effective in treating cognitive dysfunction. In recent research, Moreau and his colleages [28] asked if cognition can be enhanced via training. On the one hand, there is potential to prove the effect of intervention with applications ranging from developmental disorders to cognitive aging, dementia, and traumatic brain injury rehabilitation. On the other hand, it is difficult, because establishing clear evidence for an intervention is particularly challenging in psychology. Due to logistic shortcomings or to common difficulties in disguising the underlying hypothesis of an experiment, it is not always feasible to assure double-blind randomized controlled experiments. These limitations have important consequences for the strength of evidence in favor of an intervention [28]. Hämäläinen and Rosti-Otajärvi [29] based on rehabiliation and traning program concluded that there are positive effects of neuropsychological rehabilitation in MS.

Lizanne Evavan den Akker and her colleagues [30] tested short and long-term effects of cognitive behavioral therapy (CBT) for the treatment of MS-related fatigue. They performed a meta-analysis of the effectiveness of CBT for fatigue in patients with MS. The results indicated a moderately positive short-term effect of CBT for the treatment of fatigue in patients with MS. However, this effect declined after cessation of treatment. The authors suggested that since the short-term effect of CBT on MS-related fatigue is positive, more research is needed to develop interventions that maintain these short-term effects for the long term.

Regarding the nature of the effect obtained following cognitive therapy, work by Penner et al. [31] used neuroimaging techniques to study the effects of cognitive rehabilitation in MS including task-based fMRI across multiple realms of cognition (e.g, executive functioning, attention, and processing speed). MS patients were examined using fMRI before and after cognitive practice in attentional tasks. The results of the study indicated that after the practice, there was an increase in activation that was more pronounced in the parietal and frontal areas, but the degree of activation was not correlated with an improvement in the performance of tasks. Apparently, performance improvement depends on the capacity of the brain to establish new functional pathways.

Hayes and his colleagues [31] reviewed 13 studies with 839 participants involving various types of fall interventions, most comparing an exercise intervention with no intervention or two or more fall prevention interventions. They tried to explore whether 1. people with multiple sclerosis (MS) who received interventions to reduce falls show better fall outcomes than those who received no treatment?2. different types of falls interventions result in different outcomes for people with MS. Based on the results, they concluded that "there is some evidence in favor of exercise interventions for the improvement of balance function and mobility. However, this must be interpreted with caution as the results represent data from a small number of studies." Looking at the whole picture, we require a science of cognitive rehabilitation capable of yielding high levels of evidence. Toward this end, theoretical models of MS-related cognitive dysfunction and ways to identify mechanisms of action to treat deficits must be developed. Finally, standards for a priori reporting of methods must be upheld for cognitive rehabilitation, including greater transparency for outcomes. In this regard, cognitive rehabilitation researchers are directed to Simons et al. [32] for a thorough discussion of essential guidelines for the conduct of high-quality cognitive intervention trials.

5. Conclusions

Several neurological disorders have a positive association with MCI cognitive deficits. This chapter reviews this association in the case of multiple sclerosis (MS), covering MS subtypes and staging, clinical and imaging assessments, and therapeutic options. MS is invariably progressive, though mild symptoms may persist for variable intervals, a fact of notable interest to patient and clinician alike. The chapter's focus on high-level cognitive function and memory-related deficits affords a unique perspective not often found in MS research with an exploration of MS-specific, memory impairments that, tragically, occur at all MS stages. The discussion of the evolution of MS with its consideration of the extent and character of these impairments as a function of stage provides a valuable backdrop against which to distill clinical diagnosis. MS subjects, as noted, can display MS-specific sets of deficits, [normal performance in non-intentional learning tasks and poor performance in tests of intentional learning; the demonstration of relatively normal short-term memory functions, while having difficulties in recollection of long-term information]. Based on these unique footprints, this chapter makes the inference that the implicit learning disorder observed in MS patients suffering from cognitive decline is due to a disconnection between the cortical regions and subcortical structures, a point of interest for targeting causal factors. It was proven that in multiple sclerosis (MS), there are physical and mental comorbidities, and adverse health factors such as smoking and obesity are common and can affect the disease. These comorbid diseases and lifestyle factors affect clinical manifestation, the disability progression, and health-related quality of life [7]. People with MS can benefit from maintaining a healthy weight, keeping up regular exercise, getting enough sleep, and staying psychologically well. This brain-healthy lifestyle could protect against further progression of MS. This chapter recommends that numerous clinical batteries can be expected to facilitate the choice of batteries optimally suited to the MS subject. These recommendations should be separate but related to and joined to the recommendation of Langdon et al. [33], for a brief International Cognitive Assessment for Multiple Sclerosis that will take into account the caveats and the comorbidities mentioned.

Author details

Raphiq Ibrahim
Edmond J. Safra Brain Research Center for the Study of Learning Disabilities, University of Haifa, Israel

*Address all correspondence to: raphiq@psy.haifa.ac.il

References

[1] Ibrahim R. Language and cognitive impairments associated with encephalitis. In: Hayasaka D, editor. Pathogenesis of Encephalitis. London, UK, Rijeka, Croatia: InTech; 2011. pp. 61-68

[2] Benedict RH, Walton MK. Evaluating cognitive outcome measures for MS clinical trials: What is a clinically meaningful change? Multiple Sclerosis. 2012;**18**:1673-1679

[3] Koutsouraki E, Kalatha T, Grosi E, Koukoulidis T, Michmizos D. Cognotove decline in multiple sclerosis patients. Journal of Nuclear Medicine. 2019;**22**:75-81

[4] Lublin FD, Reingold SC. Defining the clinical course of multiple sclerosis: Results of an international survey. Neurology. 1996;**46**:907-911

[5] Lublin FD, Baier M, Cutter G. Effect of relapses on development of residual deficit in multiple sclerosis. Neurology. 2003;**61**:1528-1532

[6] Rao SM, Leo GJ, Bernardin L, Unverzagt F. Cognitive dysfunction in multiple sclerosis: Frequency, patterns, and prediction. Neurology. 1991;**4**:685-691

[7] Marrie RA, Horwitz RI. Emerging effects of comorbidities on multiple sclerosis. The Lancet Neurology. 2010;**9**:820-828

[8] Campbell J, Rashid W, Cercignani M, Langdon D. Cognitive impairment among patients with multiple sclerosis: Associations with employment and quality of life. Postgraduate Medical Journal. 2017;**93**(1097):143-147

[9] Rao SM, Grafman J, DiGiulio D, Mittenberg W, Bernardin L, Leo GJ, et al. Memory dysfunction in multiple sclerosis: Its relation to working memory, semantic encoding, and implicit learning. Neuropsychology. 1993;**7**(3):364-374

[10] Ron MA, Callanan MM, Warrington EK. Cognitive abnormalities in multiple sclerosis: A psychometric and MRI study. Psychological Medicine. 1991;**21**(1):59-68

[11] Gaudino E, Donoffio N, DeLuca J, Diamond BJ. Acomparison of memory performance in relapsing-remitting, primary-progressive and secondary progressive multiple sclerosis. Neuropsychiatry, Neuropsychology, and Behavioral Neurology. 2001;**14**:32-44

[12] Seinela A, Hamalainen P, Koivisto M, Ruutianen J. Conscious and unconscious uses of memory in multiple sclerosis. Journal of Neurological Sciences. 2002;**198**:79-85

[13] Grafman J, Rao SM, Bernardin L, y Leo GJ. Automatic memory processes in patients with multiple sclerosis. Archives of Neurology. 1991;**48**:1072-1075

[14] Kenealy PM, Beaumont JG, Lintern TC, Murell RC. Autobiografical memory in advanced multiple sclerosis: Assessment of episodic and personal semantic memory across three time spans. Journal of International Neuropsychology Society. 2002;**8**:855-860

[15] De Sonneville LMJ, Boringa JB, Reuling IEW, Lazeron RHC, Adèr HJ, Polman CH. Information processing characteristics in subtypes of multiple sclerosis. Neuropsychologia. 2002;**40**:1751-1765

[16] Rao SM, Losinski G, Mourany L, et al. Processing speed test: Validation of a self-administered, iPad-based tool

for screening cognitive dysfunction in a clinic setting. Multiple Sclerosis. 2017;**23**:1929-1937

[17] Fisk JD, Archibald CJ. Limitations of the Paced Auditory Serial Addition Test (PASAT) as a measure of working memory in patients with multiple sclerosis. Journal of the International Neuropsychological Society. 2001;7:363-372

[18] Laatu S, Revonsuo A, Hamalainen P, et al. Visual object recognition in multiple sclerosis. Journal of the Neurological Sciences. 2001;**185**:77-88

[19] Stephan KE, Friston KJ. Analyzing effective connectivity with functional magnetic resonance imaging. Wiley Interdisciplinary Reviews: Cognitive Science. 2010;**1**:446-459

[20] Friston KJ et al. Granger causality revisited. NeuroImage. 2014;**101**:796-808

[21] Havlicek M et al. Physiologically informed dynamic causal modeling of fMRI data. NeuroImage. 2015;**122**:355-372

[22] Ross DT, Ebner FF. Thalamic retrograde degeneration following cortical injury: An excitotoxic process? Neuroscience. 1990;**35**(3):525-550

[23] Colasanti A, Guo Q, Giannetti P, et al. Hippocampal neuroinflammation, functional connectivity, and depressive symptoms in multiple sclerosis. Biological Psychiatry. 2016;**80**:62-72

[24] Veréb D, Kovács MA, Kocsis K, Tóth E, Bozsik B, Király A, et al. Functional connectivity lateralization shift of resting state networks is linked to visuospatial memory and white matter microstructure in relapsing-remitting. Multiple Sclerosis. 2022;**35**(2):268-275

[25] Huber SJ, Bornstein RA, Rammohan KW, Christy JA, Chakeres DW, McGhee RB. Magnetic resonance imaging correlates of neuropsychological impairment in multiple sclerosis. Journal of Neuropsychiatry and Clinical Neurosciences. 1992;**4**:152-158

[26] Staffen W, Mair A, Zauner H, et al. Cognitive function and fMRI in patients with multiple sclerosis: Evidence for compensatory cortical activation during an attention task. Brain. 2002;**125**:1275-1282

[27] Zivadinov R, Sepcic J, Nasuelli D, De Masi R, et al. A longitudinal study of brain atrophy and cognitive disturbances in the early phase of relapsing-remitting multiple sclerosis. Journal of Neurology, Neurosurgery, and Psychiatry. 2001;**70**(6):773-780

[28] Moreau D, Kirk IJ, Waldie KE. Seven Pervasive Statistical Flaws in Cognitive Training Interventions. Frontiers in Human *Neuroscience*. 2016;**10**:153

[29] Hämäläinen P, Rosti-Otajärvi E. Is neuropsychological rehabilitation effective in multiple sclerosis? Neurodegenerative Disease Management. 2014;**4**:147-154

[30] den Akker LE, Beckerman H, Hubertine E, Catharine CI, Eijssen JM, Dekker J, et al. Effectiveness of cognitive behavioral therapy for the treatment of fatigue in patients with multiple sclerosis: A systematic review and meta-analysis. Journal of Psychosomatic Research. 2016;**90**:33-42

[31] Hayes S, Galvin R, Kennedy C, Finlayson M, McGuigan C, Walsh CD, et al. Interventions for preventing falls in people with multiple sclerosis. Cochrane Database of Systematic Reviews. 2019;**11**

[32] Simons AD, Padesky CA, Montemarano J, Lewis CC, Murakami J,

Lamb K, et al. Training and dissemination of cognitive behavior therapy for depression in adults: A preliminary examination of therapist competence and client outcomes. Journal of Consulting and Clinical Psychology. 2010;**78**(5):751-756

[33] Langdon DW, Amato MP, Boringa J, et al. Recommendations for a Brief International Cognitive Assessment for Multiple Sclerosis (BICAMS). Multiple Sclerosis. 2012;**18**:891-898

Chapter 7

Innate Immunopathological Mechanisms in Multiple Sclerosis

Abhishek Shastri, Iesha Singh and Uday Kishore

Abstract

Multiple sclerosis (MS) is a progressive disease that affects the central nervous system. The core features of MS are demyelination and inflammation. Demyelination refers to degeneration of myelin that covers the neurons and helps facilitate neuronal impulses. Loss of myelin results in inability to conduct impulses, which causes core symptoms of MS such as unsteadiness, weakness, numbness, and tingling. Inflammation is observed at the site of demyelination in the form of scars, and hence, the term sclerosis. Innate immunity is that part of the immune system that is present from birth. Over the years, adaptive immunity has been extensively studied with respect to MS in human and experimental disease models. However, recent evidence has increasingly pointed to significant involvement of innate immune mechanisms in the pathogenesis of MS. This chapter reviews the latest evidence regarding innate immune components such as blood–brain barrier, microglial cells, and complement system, and their role in MS pathogenesis.

Keywords: innate immunity, complement system, neuroinflammation, multiple sclerosis, blood–brain barrier, microglia

1. Introduction

Multiple sclerosis (MS), a progressive neurological disease, is a lifelong illness. The course of the disease can be heterogenous, with reversible neurological deficits seen in clinically isolated syndrome and relapsing–remitting type MS; progressive form of MS results in chronic progression of clinical deficits, and is termed as primary progressive MS. The complexity and heterogeneity of clinical presentation make it imperative to understand the aetiopathogenesis of MS in order to help understand the disease and develop effective treatment modalities. Developing MS means a lifelong process for a person and till date, there has been no known cure for the disease.

The MS pathogenesis has traditionally been considered to be autoimmune in nature. In this regard, myelin proteins, such as myelin basic protein, myelin-associated glycoprotein, and myelin oligodendrocyte glycoprotein, have been extensively studied and used in animal models to induce paralytic and demyelinating disease resembling MS called as experimental autoimmune encephalomyelitis (EAE) [1].

Some of the immunopathological changes observed in MS include breakdown of blood–brain barrier (BBB), neuroinflammation, demyelination, gliosis, oligodendrocyte degeneration, and gliosis [2]. This chapter will focus on neuroinflammation involving innate immune components such as BBB, microglial cells, and the complement system.

2. Role of blood: brain barrier in MS

BBB is a tightly regulated barrier that is known to facilitate homeostasis of CNS allowing for controlled exchange of metabolic substances and prevent the entry of pathogens into the CNS, thereby acting as a basic first line of defense for the CNS. It is formed of cerebral endothelial cells tightly joined to each other and dynamically interacting with astrocytes, pericytes, and basement membrane (together known as neurovascular unit) [3]. In MS, BBB has been shown to be compromised as the first sign of disease pathogenesis, preceding infiltration of immune cells into CNS and demyelination. Some of the core changes observed include BBB disruption, perivascular astrogliosis, and increased expression of endothelial cell adhesion molecules [4]. Neuroimaging studies have revealed that gadolinium (a marker for detecting BBB disruption) is seen with active inflammation in MS lesions and is a key diagnostic sign. In fact, BBB disruption has now been observed in normal-appearing white matter before enhancing lesions. Furthermore, in few patients, optic neuritis can be the earliest sign of MS, and permeability of BBB has been shown to be predictive in progression from optic neuritis to MS [5]. This highlights the heterogeneity involved in initial MS pathogenesis in the context of BBB breakdown. Another interesting feature observed is that during the initial phases of illness, that is, in the first year of the disease, gadolinium-positive lesions are observed on MRI scans indicative of high permeability of BBB, and this is associated with frequent relapses. As time goes by, the course of illness changes to that of less BBB breakdown and more of an intrinsic CNS inflammation, which occurs as a result of the influx of leucocytes and other adaptive immune components as a part of autoimmune processes, adding to the complexity in devising effective disease management strategies [6].

Several metabolic changes are observed in BBB of MS patients. In vitro studies using sera from relapsing–remitting type MS patients have shown that BBB undergoes significant metabolic dysfunction such as reduced expression of proteins, such as occludin and cadherin, which maintain junctional integrity, reduced glycolysis in cells, and increased pro-inflammatory status indicated by higher release of reactive oxygen species from endothelial cells. These changes cause increased BBB permeability and lead to increased susceptibility to disease progression [7].

One of the early features of increased permeability of BBB in MS is infiltration of neutrophils into the CNS. Neutrophils play an important role in the MS pathogenesis and in EAE models. MS patients show higher peripheral neutrophil count as compared to healthy controls [8]. In EAE mice model, neutrophils have been shown to increase in number before and during the onset of clinical EAE and accumulate in the meninges [9, 10]. Depletion of neutrophils in EAE mice using antibody against neutrophils, prior to disease onset has been found to inhibit the early stages of disease and future relapses, with prevention of breakdown of BBB considered to be a significant factor in this process [11–13]. Migration of neutrophils across the BBB has been found to induce production of interleukin (IL)1β, which are known to, leads to increased production of Granulocyte Macrophage Colony-stimulating factor (known to promote expansion and enhance release of bone marrow-derived neutrophils), thereby further exaggerating neuroinflammation in EAE [14, 15]. Activated microglia and macrophages are known to produce enzymes such as myeloperoxidase (MPO), which are known to activate and promote accumulation of neutrophils in the CNS. Postmortem brain studies of patients with MS when compared to healthy controls, show elevated MPO level which associates significantly with demyelination [16]. Neutrophils are considered to promote disruption of BBB via release of MPO; inhibition of MPO using a specific peptide called as N-acetyl lysyltyrosylcysteine amide in EAE model caused reduced migration of neutrophils to CNS, reduced breakdown of BBB, and attenuation of the EAE severity [17].

3. Role of microglia in MS

Microglia are innate immune cells of the CNS. These resident macrophages of CNS are responsible for various homeostatic functions such as synaptic pruning, secretion of neuronal growth factors, phagocytosis of cells in developing nervous system, and maintaining vascular tone of the BBB [18]. Microglial cells show 'ramified' appearance when in resting or homeostatic state surveying the CNS as an innate immune cell, while activated microglial cells tend to reveal a more 'amoeboid' appearance [18].

Microglial cells can form about 45% of the pool of macrophage-like cells in MS lesions, as measured by marker TMEM119, which is present on microglia and not on macrophages. In addition, microglia in MS lesions show reduction in specific marker P2RY12 that is expressed only in resting or homeostatic microglia and not in active microglia, thus showing presence of activated microglia in MS lesions [19]. In areas of active demyelination, microglia show proinflammatory-type phenotype, also known as M1 type polarization that is associated with neuroinflammation and neurotoxicity (characterized by markers such as CD86, CD68, p22phox, and MHC Class II antigens). Lesions of later or inactive stages are associated with microglial cells that show anti-inflammatory phenotype, also known as M2 polarization, which is associated with resolution of neuroinflammation and neuroprotection (characterized by markers such as CD206, CD163, and ferritin) [19]. Clinically, magnetic resonance imaging (MRI) is the first choice to detect focal inflammatory lesions. However, in progressive type of MS, plaques that are associated with chronic and progressive forms of disease are characterized by 'slowly evolving/expanding' type of lesions, also known as smoldering lesions that are represented by a 'rim' of microglia and macrophages, and ongoing demyelination and loss of axons [20]. To increase specificity of detecting activated microglia, positron emission tomography (PET) is done using tracers that target a specific protein called translocator protein (TSPO)[1], which is expressed on the outer mitochondrial membrane of microglia. This is considered to be a more specific marker for neuroinflammation and progression of MS, along with assessing the effects of treatment in MS [21].

Another interesting aspect of microglial involvement in MS includes its role in lipid metabolism. Triggering receptor expressed on myeloid cells 2 (TREM2) is an immunoreceptor expressed on microglia that helps in lipid metabolism and regulation of lipid transport in CNS, along with recognition of bacterial ligands such as lipopolysaccharide, cardiolipin, sulfatides, as well as physiological ligands such as low-density lipoprotein and apolipoprotein E (apoE) [22]. TREM2 and apoE metabolic pathways are crucial in microglial switching from homeostatic state to a neurodegenerative state; mutations in TREM2 are associated with increased

[1] TSPO ligands are used to target translocator protein found on outer mitochondrial membrane of microglia. This is used as a marker to observe 'real time' activation of microglia under PET scanner.

microglia-mediated neurodegeneration [23, 24]. Soluble TREM2 level in cerebrospinal fluid (CSF) has been proposed to be a useful biomarker for microglial activation in MS, as well as for assessing response to treatment in MS. Increased level of soluble TREM2 is observed in CSF of MS patients when compared to controls, which is reduced to physiological levels following treatment with natalizumab[2] [25, 26]. Postmortem histopathological studies of MS patients also show high expression of TREM2 in demyelinating lesions. Mice deficient in TREM2 show reduced microglial activation and increased accumulation of myelin debris, while antibody-dependent TREM2 activation was found to increase oligodendrocyte production, which sustains and enhances remyelination [27].

Neuroinflammation also promotes lipid peroxidation, which leads to generation of oxidized phospholipids such as oxidized phosphatidylcholines (OxPCs). OxPCs, considered to be mediators of neurodegeneration, are found in the lesions of MS [28]. In MS, OxPCs have been directly implicated in the disease pathogenesis, along with microglia and TREM2. In an elegant study, endogenous OxPCs were found to be formed in a histopathological study on MS patients brain tissue. The authors then showed that OxPCs *in vitro* are toxic to neurons and oligodendrocytes. Direct injection of proinflammatory factors such as IL-1β in EAE mice model showed OxPC deposition in spinal cord lesions, indicating a possible role of caspase-3 pathway in this mechanism. Moreover, direct injection of OxPCs into the spinal cord of mice also resulted in demyelination and loss of oligodendrocytes, while neutralization of OxPCs by antibody showed reduced neurodegeneration. Microglial cells were found to accumulate OxPCs; loss of such microglial cells were found to exacerbate neurodegeneration, thus highlighting a protective role for microglia. TREM2 was shown to directly bind OxPCs; mice lacking TREM2 showed exacerbated neurodegeneration. Thus, TREM2 can bind and clear OxPCs and help in preventing neurodegeneration [29, 30].

4. Role of complement system in MS

The complement system is a major part of the innate immunity and consists of more than 40 serum and membrane-bound proteins. There are three activating pathways, namely (i) classical pathway, which is mainly antibody-mediated with C1q being the first ligand recognition subcomponent; (ii) alternative pathway is activated spontaneously by low-level hydrolysis of C3 to C3(H_2O); (iii) lectin pathway is activated *via* mannan-binding lectin (MBL) and ficolins. Each pathway leads to the generation of target cell lysing membrane attack complex (MAC). For further information on the role of complement system in CNS physiology and pathology, see review by Shastri et al. [18]. Here, we will focus on its role in MS and possible treatment avenues.

Complement proteins, such as C4, C1-inhibitor, and properdin, have been found to be elevated in the CSF of patients with MS. Postmortem immunohistochemistry of MS tissues has shown positive staining for several complement proteins such as C1q and C3; for activation products such as C3b, C4d, MAC; and for regulators such as factor H, clusterin and C1-inhibitor. Complement activation is observed in both white and gray matter lesions, indicating a key role for

[2] Natalizumab is a humanized monoclonal antibody against α4 integrins and is an effective treatment used in relapsing–remitting type of MS. It prevents the migration of leucocytes across the blood–brain barrier.

complement system in the MS pathogenesis [31–33]. Systemic inhibition of MAC by subcutaneous administration of a specific antisense oligonucleotide specifically targeting murine C6 mRNA that blocks formation of MAC, in EAE disease model has been found to successfully limit chronic relapsing symptoms by reducing neuroinflammation and protecting from axonal and neuronal synaptic damage. The key mechanism involved reduced secretion of IL-1β [34]. Lectin pathway activity and MBL-associated serine proteases-2 plasma levels were found to be increased in MS patients' serum when compared to controls [35].

An involvement of complement system in MS is quite evident in EAE disease model studies. Mice deficient in either C3 or factor B showed significantly reduced severity of disease and protection from demyelination [36]. Another study showed an increased level of C1q and C3 in EAE mice; C3 deficiency was shown to protect mice from synaptic loss and reduced level of microglial activation [37]. In an elegant study, it was found that in patients with MS and as well as EAE animal model, significant loss of synapses occurs along with engulfment of presynaptic terminals by microglial cells associated with activation of C3. Blockage of C3 by viral overexpression of C3-inhibitor Crry restored the demyelinating function, thus indicating a key role for complement interaction with microglial cells in MS [38]. C3 levels are also increased the dentate gyrus (a key region of hippocampus involved in episodic memory) of EAE disease model, with microglial cells being the main source of C3 in the region. Inhibition of C3 function using rosmarinic acid, which blocks C3b attachment to complement-activating surface, showed reduced loss of synapses and improved memory performance in EAE mice [39]. C1q level has also been found to be increased in MS patients and EAE model. Inhibition of C1q function by knockdown of C1s subunit of C1 was found to reduce demyelination and improve neurological function in EAE mice [40].

Recent studies have assessed the usefulness of measuring complement activation as a potential biomarker for MS progression. For example, neuromyelitis optica (NMO) is another autoimmune demyelinating disorder; it can be hard to differentiate NMO from MS especially in the early stages of the disease due to similar clinical presentation. In a study that included CSF analyses of patients with MS and NMO, a statistical model involving six complement proteins namely C3, C9, factor B, C1q, factor I, and properdin was able to differentiate between MS and NMO [33]. Response gene to complement-32 (RGC32) is a molecule induced by activation of complement; RGC32 mRNA expression is significantly decreased during relapse and increased in responders to a specific treatment called as glatiramer acetate therapy. Predictive statistical model is considered to be about 90% accurate in detecting relapses and about 85% accurate in detecting response to therapy [41]. It is also worth noting that phase 3, randomized, double-blind clinical trials using eculizumab, a monoclonal antibody against C5, has been found to be significantly effective in relapse prevention in NMO [42].

As mentioned earlier, the progressive form of MS is characterized by smoldering lesions represented by microglial cells. Absinta et al. [43] identified that white matter from healthy individuals consisted of mainly oligodendrocytes, while those from MS lesions contained immune cells such as microglia, macrophages, monocytes, dendritic cells and astrocytes, along with reduced oligodendrocytes. The authors further studied microglial cells in MS lesion edges and found an increased expression of C1 complex (C1q, C1r, and C1s) genes. Further analysis of a cohort of more than a thousand MS patients revealed that complement protein risk variants (C1QA, CR1, and C3) were associated with clinically significant lesions observed on MRI scans. The authors then induced EAE in a conditionally knocked out C1q mice model that specifically ablated C1q in microglia, which attenuated microglia activation, suggesting the importance of C1q-mediated microglial activation in MS. Blocking C1q in EAE mice reduced density of microglial cells in white matter lesions [43, 44].

5. Role of other pattern-recognition receptors

Apart from complement system, a number of innate immune pattern-recognition receptors (PRRs) have also been implicated in the pathogenesis of MS. Toll-like receptors (TLRs) are type 1 membrane proteins and contain an extracellular leucine-rich domain involved in pathogen-associated molecular pattern (PAMP) recognition and a cytoplasmic Toll/IL1 receptor (TIR) domain, which is involved in signaling pathway. It is well-known that TLRs are expressed on microglia and other CNS cells such as neurons and astrocytes [18]. Upon PAMP receptor (PRR) binding with ligand, adapter protein recruitment takes place as part of the signaling pathway. Adapter proteins include myeloid differentiating factor 88 (MyD88), MyD88 adapter-like protein, TIR domain-containing adapter inducing interferon-β (TRIF), TRIF-related adapter molecule, and sterile-α and armadillo-motif- containing protein. These adapter proteins activate microglia that ultimately lead to release of chemokines and proinflammatory cytokines such as IL-1β, tumor necrosis factor α (TNFα), and IL-6 [18]. TLR2 levels are increased in the serum of MS patients. An enhanced activation of TLR2 was observed in peripheral blood mononuclear cells (PBMCs) of MS patients when stimulated with TLR2 ligand [45, 46]. In another study involving PBMCs from MS patients, a lower baseline level of TLR8 was found when compared to healthy controls, and transcriptional response of proinflammatory cytokine IL-12β was also found to be impaired in serum of MS patients [47]. TLR and MyD88 activation pathways influence adhesion molecules of BBB, thereby playing a role in BBB disruption and subsequently in MS pathogenesis [47, 48]. Furthermore, TLR4 is considered to play a dual role with its involvement in remyelination as well as demyelination processes, which remains unclear. EAE studies have shown that TLR4-deficient mice develop more severe symptoms, while other studies show that TLR4-deficient mice develop less severe symptoms [48, 49]. This discrepancy is possibly explained by the method of induction of EAE, which varied in both these studies, and a difference in using MOG peptide by Kerfoot et al. [48] as compared to MOG protein by Marta et al. [49], which show a difference in induction of B and T cell response, thereby having an impact on demyelination process. Modulation of TLR9 activity in MyD88-deficient mice was found to render it resistant to developing EAE [50].

Nucleotide-binding and oligomerization domain (NOD)-like receptors (NLRs) are intracellular PRRs and contain a central nucleotide-binding and oligomerization (NACHT) domain and C-terminal leucine-rich repeat (LRR). NLRs can be further divided based on their N-terminal component into caspase activation and recruitment domain, pyrin domain, and baculovirus inhibitor of apoptosis protein repeat, respectively, called NLRC, NLRP, and NLRB. Binding of NLR to ligand leads to a signaling process causing formation of inflammasomes and ultimately cause release of proinflammatory cytokines such as IL-1β and IL-18 [18]. Clinically, a homozygous variant of NLRP1 gene has been found to be associated with a familial type of MS [51]. Also, in MS patients who respond to treatment, NLRP3 expression is increased, as compared to those who do not respond to treatment [52]. In EAE, deficiency of NLRP3 [53] or NLRP12 [54] is associated with reduced severity of the disease. Inhibition of NLRP3 inflammasome activity was found to reduce production of IL-1β and diminish response of T-cells, thereby reducing severity of disease [55].

6. Conclusions

MS can be described as being heterogeneous in terms of clinical presentation, complexity, and progression of disease (summarized in **Figure 1**). This is largely due to numerous pathophysiological changes occurring in the patients. Adaptive immunity has been studied extensively over the years, but less emphasis had been placed on innate immune changes that occur in MS. This notion has changed, and now there is an increasing number of studies that are looking at the key role of innate immune components in the pathogenesis of MS. One of the challenges in this regard is recruitment of patients at different stages of illness and replicating such findings to arrive at a robust and reliable conclusion. Other useful aspects of studying innate immune components are to understand and establish their role in facilitating predictive,

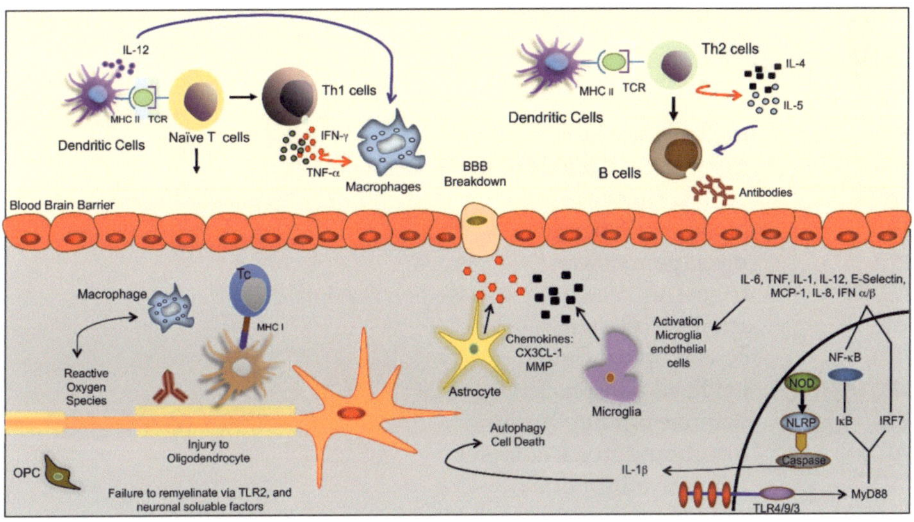

Figure 1.
Pathophysiology of multiple sclerosis: Contact in early childhood with a pathogen and other susceptibility factors, such as racial and demographic background, can elicit reactivation, triggering innate immune mechanisms via toll-like receptors (TLRs), which signal downstream through MyD88 (myeloid differentiation primary response 88) and phosphorylated IκB, allowing nuclear translocation of NF-kB and the transcription of IL-6, TNF, IL-1, IL-12, and E-selectin. IFN/transcription is signaled by TLR via IRF7 (interferon regulatory factor 7). Another significant signal is provided by NOD receptors (nucleotide-binding oligomerization domain), which are activated by potassium efflux-inducing substances such as ATP and TLR stimulation; pathogen associated molecular patterns (PAMPs) toxins, danger, or stress activate the inflammasome through nucleotide-binding oligomerization domain, leucine rich repeat and pyrin domain containing (NLRP), which forms a complex with ASC (apoptosis-associated speck-like protein containing a CARD) and caspase-1, triggering IL-1β. All of these proinflammatory cytokines and growth factors stimulate microglia and endothelial cells, upregulating the expression of adhesion molecules such as E-selectin and increasing the movement of T cells into the CNS. Matrix metallo proteases (MMP) degrade the blood–brain barrier (BBB), hence facilitating the migration of autoreactive T lymphocytes and macrophages via proinflammatory cytokines (CX3CL-1). The Th1 response induced by IL-12 and IFN-stimulates macrophages, activating CD8⁺ T cells. Th2 response mediated by IL-6 primarily increases B cell maturation and autoantibody production. Cytotoxic oligodendrocyte destruction results in myelin loss and axon exposure to reactive oxygen species that delay or stop action potentials and the formation of neurological symptoms. OPCs (oligodendrocyte precursor cells) are intended to remyelinate these lesions, but neuronal factors such as TLR2 impede their migration.

diagnostic, and prognostic markers in the clinical setting. Further understanding of innate immune components in MS would also aid future research using animal or experimental models that incorporates innate immune aspects as a part of studies in order to justify the heterogenous nature of MS pathophysiology.

In this regard, considerable progress has been made in establishing role of BBB, PRRs, and microglial cells. There is considerable evidence to suggest that BBB breakdown is a key stage in MS pathogenesis, along with complement activation. Experimental studies have been successful in attenuating severity of MS by blocking activated complement proteins. More evidence continues to accumulate to highlight the possible protective role of microglial cells in association with lipid metabolism and myelination. There is still a long way to go in terms of developing clinically useful biomarkers, better research disease models, and effective and safer treatment strategies to benefit patients and improve their overall quality of life.

Conflict of interest

The authors declare no conflict of interest.

Abbreviations

MS	multiple sclerosis
EAE	experimental autoimmune encephalomyelitis
CNS	central nervous system
BBB	blood–brain barrier
MPO	myeloperoxidase
TREM2	triggering receptor expressed on myeloid cells 2
apoE	apolipoprotein E
CSF	cerebrospinal fluid
OxPC	oxidized phosphatidylcholine
MBL	mannan binding lectin
MAC	membrane attack complex
NMO	neuromyelitis optica
TLR	toll-like receptor
MyD88	myeloid differentiating factor 88
TRIF	TIR domain-containing adapter inducing interferon-β
NOD	nucleotide-binding and oligomerization domain
NLR	NOD-like receptor

Author details

Abhishek Shastri[1*], Iesha Singh[2] and Uday Kishore[3]

1 Central and North West London NHS Foundation Trust, London, United Kingdom

2 Imperial College London, London, United Kingdom

3 Department of Veterinary Medicine, UAE University, Al Ain, United Arab Emirates

*Address all correspondence to: abhishek.shastri@nhs.net

References

[1] Glatigny S, Bettelli E. Experimental Autoimmune Encephalomyelitis (EAE) as animal models of multiple sclerosis (MS). Cold Spring Harbor Perspective Medicine. 2018;**8**(11):1101

[2] Baecher-Allan C, Kaskow BJ, Weiner HL. Multiple sclerosis: Mechanisms and immunotherapy. Neuron. 2018;**97**(4):742-768

[3] Iadecola C. The neurovascular unit coming of age: A journey through neurovascular coupling in health and disease. Neuron. 2017;**96**(1):17-42

[4] Alvarez JI, Saint-Laurent O, Godschalk A, Terouz S, Briels C, Larouche S, et al. Focal disturbances in the blood-brain barrier are associated with formation of neuroinflammatory lesions. Neurobiology of Disease. 2015;**74**:14-24

[5] Cramer SP, Modvig S, Simonsen HJ, Frederiksen JL, Larsson HB. Permeability of the blood-brain barrier predicts conversion from optic neuritis to multiple sclerosis. Brain. 2015;**138**(Pt 9):2571-2583

[6] Spencer JI, Bell JS, DeLuca GC. Vascular pathology in multiple sclerosis: Reframing pathogenesis around the blood-brain barrier. Journal of Neurology, Neurosurgery, and Psychiatry. 2018;**89**(1):42-52

[7] Sheikh MH, Henson SM, Loiola RA, Mercurio S, Colamatteo A, Maniscalco GT, et al. Immuno-metabolic impact of the multiple sclerosis patients' sera on endothelial cells of the blood-brain barrier. Journal of Neuroinflammation. 2020;**17**(1):153

[8] Akaishi T, Misu T, Fujihara K, Nakaya N, Nakamura T, Kogure M, et al. White blood cell count profiles in multiple sclerosis during attacks before the initiation of acute and chronic treatments. Scientific Reports. 2021;**11**(1):22357

[9] Rumble JM, Huber AK, Krishnamoorthy G, Srinivasan A, Giles DA, Zhang X, et al. Neutrophil-related factors as biomarkers in EAE and MS. The Journal of Experimental Medicine. 2015;**212**(1):23-35

[10] Christy AL, Walker ME, Hessner MJ, Brown MA. Mast cell activation and neutrophil recruitment promotes early and robust inflammation in the meninges in EAE. Journal of Autoimmunity. 2013;**42**:50-61

[11] McColl SR, Staykova MA, Wozniak A, Fordham S, Bruce J, Willenborg DO. Treatment with anti-granulocyte antibodies inhibits the effector phase of experimental autoimmune encephalomyelitis. Journal of Immunology. 1998;**161**(11):6421-6426

[12] Carlson T, Kroenke M, Rao P, Lane TE, Segal B. The Th17-ELR+ CXC chemokine pathway is essential for the development of central nervous system autoimmune disease. The Journal of Experimental Medicine. 2008;**205**(4):811-823

[13] Aube B, Levesque SA, Pare A, Chamma E, Kebir H, Gorina R, et al. Neutrophils mediate blood-spinal cord barrier disruption in demyelinating neuroinflammatory diseases. Journal of Immunology. 2014;**193**(5):2438-2454

[14] Levesque SA, Pare A, Mailhot B, Bellver-Landete V, Kebir H, Lecuyer MA, et al. Myeloid cell transmigration across the CNS vasculature triggers

IL-1beta-driven neuroinflammation during autoimmune encephalomyelitis in mice. The Journal of Experimental Medicine. 2016;**213**(6):929-949

[15] De Bondt M, Hellings N, Opdenakker G, Struyf S. Neutrophils: Underestimated players in the pathogenesis of multiple sclerosis (MS). International Journal of Molecular Sciences. 2020;**21**(12):3390. DOI: 10.3390/ijms21124558

[16] Gray E, Thomas TL, Betmouni S, Scolding N, Love S. Elevated myeloperoxidase activity in white matter in multiple sclerosis. Neuroscience Letters. 2008;**444**(2):195-198

[17] Zhang H, Ray A, Miller NM, Hartwig D, Pritchard KA, Dittel BN. Inhibition of myeloperoxidase at the peak of experimental autoimmune encephalomyelitis restores blood-brain barrier integrity and ameliorates disease severity. Journal of Neurochemistry. 2016;**136**(4):826-836

[18] Shastri A, Bonifati DM, Kishore U. Innate immunity and neuroinflammation. Mediators of Inflammation. 2013;**2013**:342931

[19] Zrzavy T, Hametner S, Wimmer I, Butovsky O, Weiner HL, Lassmann H. Loss of 'homeostatic' microglia and patterns of their activation in active multiple sclerosis. Brain. 2017;**140**(7):1900-1913

[20] Filippi M, Preziosa P, Banwell BL, Barkhof F, Ciccarelli O, De Stefano N, et al. Assessment of lesions on magnetic resonance imaging in multiple sclerosis: Practical guidelines. Brain. 2019;**142**(7):1858-1875

[21] Airas L, Rissanen E, Rinne J. Imaging of microglial activation in MS using PET: Research use and potential future clinical application. Multiple Sclerosis. 2017;**23**(4):496-504

[22] Deczkowska A, Weiner A, Amit I. The physiology, pathology, and potential therapeutic applications of the TREM2 Signaling pathway. Cell. 2020;**181**(6):1207-1217

[23] Kleinberger G, Yamanishi Y, Suarez-Calvet M, Czirr E, Lohmann E, Cuyvers E, et al. TREM2 mutations implicated in neurodegeneration impair cell surface transport and phagocytosis. Science Translational Medicine. 2014;**6**(243):243ra86

[24] Jonsson T, Stefansson H, Steinberg S, Jonsdottir I, Jonsson PV, Snaedal J, et al. Variant of TREM2 associated with the risk of Alzheimer's disease. The New England Journal of Medicine. 2013;**368**(2):107-116

[25] Piccio L, Buonsanti C, Cella M, Tassi I, Schmidt RE, Fenoglio C, et al. Identification of soluble TREM-2 in the cerebrospinal fluid and its association with multiple sclerosis and CNS inflammation. Brain. 2008;**131**(Pt 11):3081-3091

[26] Ohrfelt A, Axelsson M, Malmestrom C, Novakova L, Heslegrave A, Blennow K, et al. Soluble TREM-2 in cerebrospinal fluid from patients with multiple sclerosis treated with natalizumab or mitoxantrone. Multiple Sclerosis. 2016;**22**(12):1587-1595

[27] Cignarella F, Filipello F, Bollman B, Cantoni C, Locca A, Mikesell R, et al. TREM2 activation on microglia promotes myelin debris clearance and remyelination in a model of multiple sclerosis. Acta Neuropathologica. 2020;**140**(4):513-534

[28] Dong Y, Yong VW. Oxidized phospholipids as novel mediators

of neurodegeneration. Trends in Neurosciences. 2022;**45**(6):419-429

[29] Dong Y, D'Mello C, Pinsky W, Lozinski BM, Kaushik DK, Ghorbani S, et al. Oxidized phosphatidylcholines found in multiple sclerosis lesions mediate neurodegeneration and are neutralized by microglia. Nature Neuroscience. 2021;**24**(4):489-503

[30] Monroe KM, Di Paolo G. Microglia clean up toxic lipids in multiple sclerosis. Nature Neuroscience. 2021;**24**(4):451-452

[31] Ingram G, Loveless S, Howell OW, Hakobyan S, Dancey B, Harris CL, et al. Complement activation in multiple sclerosis plaques: An immunohistochemical analysis. Acta Neuropathologica Communications. 2014;**2014**:53

[32] Watkins LM, Neal JW, Loveless S, Michailidou I, Ramaglia V, Rees MI, et al. Complement is activated in progressive multiple sclerosis cortical grey matter lesions. Journal of Neuroinflammation. 2016;**13**(1):161

[33] Zelek WM, Fathalla D, Morgan A, Touchard S, Loveless S, Tallantyre E, et al. Cerebrospinal fluid complement system biomarkers in demyelinating disease. Multiple Sclerosis. 2020;**26**(14):1929-1937

[34] Michailidou I, Jongejan A, Vreijling JP, Georgakopoulou T, de Wissel MB, Wolterman RA, et al. Systemic inhibition of the membrane attack complex impedes neuroinflammation in chronic relapsing experimental autoimmune encephalomyelitis. Acta Neuropathologica Communications. 2018;**6**(1):36

[35] Kwok JY, Vaida F, Augst RM, Yu DY, Singh KK. Mannose binding lectin mediated complement pathway in multiple sclerosis. Journal of Neuroimmunology. 2011;**239**(1-2):98-100

[36] Nataf S, Carroll SL, Wetsel RA, Szalai AJ, Barnum SR. Attenuation of experimental autoimmune demyelination in complement-deficient mice. Journal of Immunology. 2000;**165**(10):5867-5873

[37] Hammond JW, Bellizzi MJ, Ware C, Qiu WQ, Saminathan P, Li H, et al. Complement-dependent synapse loss and microgliosis in a mouse model of multiple sclerosis. Brain, Behavior, and Immunity. 2020;**87**:739-750

[38] Werneburg S, Jung J, Kunjamma RB, Ha SK, Luciano NJ, Willis CM, et al. Targeted complement inhibition at synapses prevents microglial synaptic engulfment and synapse loss in demyelinating disease. Immunity. 2020;**52**(1):167-182.e7

[39] Bourel J, Planche V, Dubourdieu N, Oliveira A, Sere A, Ducourneau EG, et al. Complement C3 mediates early hippocampal neurodegeneration and memory impairment in experimental multiple sclerosis. Neurobiology of Disease. 2021;**160**:105533

[40] Gao Z, Zhang C, Feng Z, Liu Z, Yang Y, Yang K, et al. C1q inhibits differentiation of oligodendrocyte progenitor cells via Wnt/beta-catenin signaling activation in a cuprizone-induced mouse model of multiple sclerosis. Experimental Neurology. 2022;**348**:113947

[41] Tatomir A, Talpos-Caia A, Anselmo F, Kruszewski AM, Boodhoo D, Rus V, et al. The complement system as a biomarker of disease activity and response to treatment in multiple sclerosis. Immunologic Research. 2017;**65**(6):1103-1109

[42] Pittock SJ, Berthele A, Fujihara K, Kim HJ, Levy M, Palace J, et al. Eculizumab in Aquaporin-4-positive Neuromyelitis Optica Spectrum disorder. The New England Journal of Medicine. 2019;**381**(7):614-625

[43] Absinta M, Maric D, Gharagozloo M, Garton T, Smith MD, Jin J, et al. A lymphocyte-microglia-astrocyte axis in chronic active multiple sclerosis. Nature. 2021;**597**(7878):709-714

[44] Kingwell K. Exploring new frontiers in multiple sclerosis. Nature Reviews. Drug Discovery. 2021;**20**(11):815

[45] Hossain MJ, Morandi E, Tanasescu R, Frakich N, Caldano M, Onion D, et al. The soluble form of toll-like receptor 2 is elevated in serum of multiple sclerosis patients: A novel potential disease biomarker. Frontiers in Immunology. 2018;**14**(9):457

[46] Fujiwara M, Anstadt EJ, Flynn B, Morse K, Ng C, Paczkowski P, et al. Enhanced TLR2 responses in multiple sclerosis. Clinical and Experimental Immunology. 2018;**193**(3):313-326

[47] Johnson TP, Tyagi R, Patel K, Schiess N, Calabresi PA, Nath A. Impaired toll-like receptor 8 signaling in multiple sclerosis. Journal of Neuroinflammation. 2013;**10**:74

[48] Kerfoot SM, Long EM, Hickey MJ, Andonegui G, Lapointe BM, Zanardo RCO, et al. TLR4 contributes to disease-inducing mechanisms resulting in central nervous system autoimmune disease. Journal of Immunology. 2004;**173**(11):7070-7071

[49] Marta M, Andersson A, Isakkson M, Kampe O, Lobell A. Unexpected regulatory roles of TLR4 and TLR9 in experimental autoimmune encephalomyelitis. European Journal of Immunology. 2008;**38**(2):565-575

[50] Prinz M, Garbe F, Schmidt H, Mildner A, Gutcher I, Wolter K, et al. Innate immunity mediated by TLR9 modulates pathogenicity in an animal model of multiple sclerosis. The Journal of Clinical Investigation. 2006;**116**(2):456-464

[51] Maver A, Lavtar P, Ristic S, Stopinsek S, Simcic S, Hocevar K, et al. Identification of rare genetic variation of NLRP1 gene in familial multiple sclerosis. Scientific Reports. 2017;7(1):3715

[52] Malhotra S, Rio J, Urcelay E, Nurtdinov R, Bustamante MF, Fernandez O, et al. NLRP3 inflammasome is associated with the response to IFN-beta in patients with multiple sclerosis. Brain. 2015;**138**(Pt 3):644-652

[53] Gris D, Ye Z, Iocca HA, Wen H, Craven RR, Gris P, et al. NLRP3 plays a critical role in the development of experimental autoimmune encephalomyelitis by mediating Th1 and Th17 responses. Journal of Immunology. 2010;**185**(2):974-981

[54] Lukens JR, Gurung P, Shaw PJ, Barr MJ, Zaki MH, Brown SA, et al. The NLRP12 sensor negatively regulates autoinflammatory disease by modulating Interleukin-4 production in T cells. Immunity. 2015;**42**(4):654-664

[55] Coll RC, Robertson AA, Chae JJ, Higgins SC, Munoz-Planillo R, Inserra MC, et al. A small-molecule inhibitor of the NLRP3 inflammasome for the treatment of inflammatory diseases. Nature Medicine. 2015;**21**(3):248-255